D0758459

MEGA-NUTRITION

MEGA-NUTRITION

The New Prescription
for Maximum
Health, Energy, and Longevity

Richard A. Kunin, M.D.

A John L. Hochmann Book

McGraw-Hill Book Company

New York   St. Louis   San Francisco
Düsseldorf   Mexico   Toronto

This book is not intended to replace the services of a physician. Any application of the recommendations set forth in the following pages is at the reader's discretion and sole risk.

Copyright © 1980 by Richard A. Kunin, M.D.

All rights reserved.

Printed in the United States of America.
No part of this publication may be reproduced, stored in a retrieval system, or transmitted, in any form or by any means, electronic, mechanical, photocopying, recording, or otherwise, without the prior written permission of the publisher.

To ABRAM HOFFER,
a great clinician, teacher, and humanitarian,
who had the courage, virtually alone,
to pioneer the cause of nutritional medicine
twenty years before orthomolecular principles were understood,
this book is respectfully dedicated.

ACKNOWLEDGMENTS I would like to show my appreciation to several people who have helped make this book possible: Edmond G. Addeo for invaluable research on the project; Jovita Addeo and Monica Kuehner for manuscript preparation; Robert Burger for the original impetus and writing; and scores of patients, *who are anonymous in this book,* for the support they have given me in my work.

Contents

1
The Nutrition Prescription

About ten years ago, a number of American doctors, working independently, began a quiet revolution in medical practice that challenged the foundations of health care as we then knew it. I was fortunate to be among these physicians. I was able to contribute original research and clinical observations to the understanding of nutritional deficiencies underlying mental disorders and disease. We were a diverse group, working in a variety of fields and under no unified banner. In broad terms, it could be said that we were dealing in preventive medicine. Linus Pauling coined the more specific term "orthomolecular medicine" and the word literally says it all: the right ("ortho") concentration of molecules, normally present in the body, for each bodily function. I have used the same prefix "ortho" to describe the dietary program that I consider to be the logical extension of this principle: the orthocarbohydrate diet, a method for determining the correct level of carbohydrates for each person's metabolism to increase one's feelings of good health and energy level, and even to extend one's life.

No matter what the name or field of practice, however, it soon became clear that we had a common cause and a unifying focus. We were concerned with the nutritional basis of health care *at the subclinical level*.

History will show, I believe, that this change of focus in medicine is more significant for health care than the discovery of antibiotics. Today, orthomolecular medicine is represented by a strong medical association and several regional societies, and our techniques of diagnosis and treatment are well understood and are gaining wide acceptance. But we are still a long way from affecting the general practice of medicine.

By whatever name, the "nutrition-prescription" movement is not a cult, a splinter element, nor a saboteur in modern medicine, but a new direction toward which all of medicine is moving.

In this country we have created a convenient category to segregate health-conscious, nutrition-conscious people from the rest of the populace: we call them "food faddists." We have a separate section in our bookstores to accommodate their interest; we have health food stores to cater to them. This is why, I'm afraid, so much of the message of modern nutrition is lost. We hear about such things as macrobiotics, fruitarianism, ovo-lacto vegetarianism, mucusless diets, and if they don't immediately attract us, we ignore them. Though I believe each of these movements has its points, I am more interested in what, collectively, they tell us about the whole picture. For I believe that human life is too complex and its history too full for any single, extreme dietary program to be of universal value.

When I say that I prescribe nutrition, on the other hand, I don't mean anything as vague as that I believe food is more important than drugs, or patients should learn to take care of themselves. That's the other extreme of food cultism. I prescribe nutrition for its demonstrable benefits, for its specific effects in specific circumstances, and for its superiority to drugs and other therapies in these circumstances as shown in all three forms of scientific evidence: clinical, laboratory, and epidemiological.

In my enthusiasm for this new approach—new mainly in its scientific preciseness, not in its age-old wisdom—I too have searched for a name that would make it immediately intelligible to the layperson. Meganutrition is the best description of what I'm talking about.

My main concern about the term "orthomolecular" is how laypeople will react to it. They hear only about megadoses of vitamins and of exotic diets of raw foods. That translates as overdoses, excesses of whatever is good for you. But the fact is that such drastic approaches must be made *in some cases* to overcome illnesses. In this respect, vitamin C is the most obvious example: the amount that constitutes the right dose can vary not only from person to person but also from one day to the next in the same person's life.

Let no one assume that orthomolecular medicine is, by its very name, inimical to traditional practice. I may question many approaches of traditional medicine, but I am certainly not trying to debunk it across the board. In one of my specialties, psychotherapy, I was the first to point out, as long ago as 1975, that the nutritional approach met all of the standards of a true psychotherapy. Orthomolecular medicine offers these therapeutic criteria:

1. It gives patients an explanation of their illness.
2. It offers something to do about it (which is even more important).
3. It challenges them to take responsibility for their own self-care.

The orthomolecular approach prescribes vitamins; the patient must know what vitamins in what proportions. Without the patient's understanding of the importance of vitamins, treatment could not possibly be maintained.

Undeniably, however, I feel that the emphasis on self-care throughout our society (self-medication, biofeedback, even grooming) is best exemplified in *dietary self-care*. The medical profession has come to a turning point on this issue. The cost of medical care administered like a mechanic to an automobile has become prohibitive. We are waking up to the fact that technology may not be as responsible for the lowering of the death rate as the dramatic stories in the popular media may imply. Dr. Eric J. Cassell, clinical professor of public health at Cornell University Medical College, writes in his book *The Healer's Art:*

> Since the common infectious scourges of the past have disappeared more or less simultaneously with the growth and development of modern medicine and its technical wizardry, it is commonly believed that the dramatic improvement in the health of our society was brought about by the achievements of physicians and medical science. By and large, however, this is not true.

Widespread improvements in sanitation and in the general conditions of living have made a decided impact on the spread of infectious diseases. But the emergence of a health-conscious society has had an even greater influence on the control of chronic conditions. The two most obvious examples of the layperson's involvement with health are the aerobics movement and the anti-sugar crusade. I use those words advisedly:

it has taken "movements" and "crusades" to wake people up to the notion that doctors and hospitals don't prevent disease—they discover it and treat it. And frequently not early enough, and sometimes not too terribly well.

If we had the vantage point of fifty years from now, we could see a pattern developing in this century that would help explain why the message of clinical nutrition has taken so long to come into its own. Because the early pioneers in this field—Royal Lee, Carlton Fredericks, Seale Harris, and Adelle Davis—were in a sense ahead of their time, we have had to rediscover nutrition. In the 1920s and '30s, when traditional medicine was making great scientific strides, the nutritionists lacked the evidence to support their case. They were not simply clever dreamers, but their research was overshadowed by the headline-grabbing success of drug and surgical treatment. The breakthroughs in antibiotics and new vaccines after the Second World War seemed to point to the triumphant march of medical science through every battleground of disease and illness. Because they were unable to come close to matching this convincing record, the nutritionists were relegated to the province of folklore and cultism. Even today, if a physician mentions *healing by food* at a meeting of a medical society, he or she is likely to be looked at quizzically by colleagues. *But today we have the evidence.*

Well then—now that nutrition has been rediscovered, what is its message? I can make no better start at this fundamental question than to paraphrase Dr. James C. McLester, who, more than forty years ago, summarized the focus of this book with these main points in an editorial in the *Journal of the American Medical Association:*

1. Malnutrition does not come solely from lack of vitamins, but also from a deficiency of proteins, minerals, and fats.
2. In America, nutrition is seldom complete.
3. Disease is not usually an expression of a single nutrient fault; more often it is partial and multiple, with a clinical picture correspondingly lacking in detail.

Consider for a moment what item three means. We are accustomed to thinking of medical treatment as taking a specific drug for a given illness—insulin for diabetes, penicillin for strep throat, aspirin for a headache. We experience an illness or disease only as a symptom, or a group of symptoms—we may be depressed, or have stomach pains, or have difficulty in breathing. Even if only one symptom is present, however, it may not unequivocally point to one underlying cause; diagnostics is still an art in our era of X rays, probes, and blood tests. McLester's point goes beyond this fact: the nutritional cause of a disease may also be complex. In most cases in the literature and in my experience, a variety of dietary corrections and a variety of supplements are necessary for the alleviation of even a single symptom. Don't look for a magic pill in the nutrition prescription. And just because one vitamin may be effective in a number of illnesses (vitamin C immediately comes to mind), I am not urging anyone to become a faddist by ignoring everything else in pursuit of a single aspect of nutrition.

This book is organized, in fact, in such a way as to suggest that there may very well be many treatments for a single disease and many uses for a single nutrient. So I have come at the subject from both sides: I have considered the most prevalent or serious diseases first, along with the nutritional approach to their treatment, and then the workings of the major categories of nutrients. You can pick out any subject that interests you and study it, without having missed any prerequisites in the previous chapters. Finally, I close with a prescription for a lifestyle that makes use of all the evidence in this book and includes a diet plan that can be both a diagnostic tool for your self-care and a *safe* method of determining your best weight. Yet I would hope that you will read all or most of the book purely in self-interest; for the more you know of the whole field the more you will be inclined to stay with your nutritional plan even if others may not understand.

In addition to this sort of specific approach, we will explore some larger questions of cause and effect in the nutritional-health cycle. Consider, for example, the simple question of what constitutes a scientific study. Generally a medical study consists of treating a group of patients (the larger the better, and of course with their consent) with the drug or nutrient in question, and at the same time treating a similar group with nothing (also with their consent, and usually with a similar pill that contains no active ingredients—a "placebo"). The crux of such a test lies in that simple word "similar." In Linus Pauling's and Ewan Cameron's important study of vitamin C and cancer, groups of 10 untreated patients were matched with *each* of 100 patients being treated, as similar in age, in sex, in type of tumor, and so forth. Such groups, whether one or many, are called the "control." Obviously, the better the control, the more accurate the conclusions. Knowing this, think for a minute about all the widely publicized experiments that have been conducted over the past 50 years in universities and clinics, by drug companies and by traditional medical teams. What is the most often overlooked factor in setting up their control groups? Just this: the nutritional habits and condition of their subjects. In short, conventional medicine has invalidated its tests from the very beginning.

For example, vitamin A has shown effectiveness in treating asthma. Suppose, in testing a new asthma drug, the test group just happened to eat more spinach or liver or peaches or pumpkin than the control group. The test group wouldn't have to eat much more of these foods, because they're all quite rich in vitamin A. Whether the drug worked or not, the test group would show decided improvement. The drug company would receive FDA approval if all other conditions were met, and physicians all over the country would be prescribing a worthless drug—in good faith.

I'm beginning to wonder if some of the contradictory results we see in medical studies may not be the result of failure to take the food factor into consideration.

Because the rediscovery of nutrition by the medical profession is hardly begun, we are faced with a paradox that only a bureaucrat could love. Drug companies are allowed to make health claims for their products while vitamin companies are not so allowed. It's actually illegal for a vitamin company to make health claims about its products even if true —to a doctor even!

When nutrition was removed from medical practice, we were left with only surgery, pharmacology, and psychotherapy to prevent and treat disease. That was some 40 years ago. Fortunately, in this country you can choose your own food and supplements as well as your physician. When it comes to your personal nutrition, you must think for yourself. I hope my book will help you.

2

The American Diet: Chronic Subclinical Malnutrition

Though several important books have appeared on the subject, the message of "orthomedicine" has not, I am afraid, reached the American public as more than another health fad. The very name "orthomolecular" has turned the layperson away, in spite of its preciseness. And the understandable inertia among physicians to adopt something they haven't learned in medical school has also slowed our progress. There is another factor working against the acceptance of our work, and it is a major one. I would like to deal with it head-on at the outset of this book. This roadblock is the widespread belief that good nutrition is a fact of life in America, or that at least it's within the grasp of anyone who is on a normal American diet.

Nothing could be further from the truth. The very idea of a balanced diet is a myth. First, it is based on an erroneous premise. The claim that an arbitrary mix of various food types can adequately support the health of widely varying individuals is demonstrably false. Second, a balanced diet is a practical impossibility in the society in which we live —even though it's an ideal at which to aim. The assurances we hear from the medical establishment that we can obtain all the nutrients we need from supermarket food are incessant but unsupported by the facts. Even if you studiously avoid junk food, sugar-coated cereals, and highly processed canned and packaged food products, and believe you are in good health, you may very well be undernourished. Let me tell you why.

Walking Malnutrition

Based on research and experience, I would say that the average diet in this country is a death sentence for millions of people. If you attempt to get all the vitamins and minerals you need from a normal American diet, you will not only suffer diseases needlessly, you will die several years before your time. Now, we have all heard scare stories about additives and "empty" calories. And they're all true. Unfortunately, criticisms of the American way of eating are often so general that they have lost their force with us. I would like to show you specific ways to improve your health with observable results.

I would like to demonstrate how you can be superficially healthy but walking through the day in a state of malnutrition: chronic, subclinical malnutrition.

After almost 20 years of conventional medical practice I began to explore the dozens of "small" factors in nutrition: the trace minerals, the little-known vitamins that support and regulate the myriad functions of our glands, our nervous system, our digestive system. In more than ten years of practice since then, I have treated more than 4,000 patients with orthomolecular medicine (which includes both psychiatry and nutrition). What was the state of their health and dietary habits before treatment? I decided to find out.

Since these patients came to me for specific nutritional advice and were already interested in the subject, one would have expected them to be free of the common deficiencies and they did in fact have better-than-average dietary habits. Nevertheless, when in 1975 I conducted a dietary survey of 132 of them selected at random, I found that more than half were deficient in vitamin E and a third in one or more of the B vitamins! In the latter case, the extent of the deficiencies was serious: about 30 percent below the Recommended Dietary Allowance (RDA) as defined by the Food and Nutrition Board of the National Research Council. (The RDA can also mean "Recommended *Daily* Allowance," the FDA term, but the difference is inconsequential for our purposes.) The RDA figures you see listed on many food products are merely the levels of essential nutrients estimated to be necessary to *maintain* one's health. Other deficiencies were equally surprising:

• Almost half of my sample patients were deficient in calcium and magnesium, and more than half the women lacked sufficient dietary iron. Nearly a third were deficient in iodine (as distinguished from iodized salt).

• More than half were deficient in the essential amino acid methionine, and 10 percent were low in tryptophane and phenylalinine. These are three essential amino acids out of the eight that are necessary to normal cell growth. These deficiencies are especially surprising in that the amino acids are derived from protein, and it is commonly believed that Americans have an excess of protein in their diets.

This survey, incidentally, was conducted with the help of computers—a tool that has made it possible for doctors to include nutritional analysis in their practice. This fact is becoming increasingly important for that vast majority of physicians who have not had adequate training in clinical nutrition.

In the same study, blood tests of 110 patients located 5 with low folic acid levels and another 13 who were marginally low. This B vitamin and vitamin B_{12} are important for cell growth and repair, particularly the regeneration of nucleic acids, which make up the genes contained in every cell in the body. These genes control blood-cell formation, nerve function, formation of hormones and neurohormones, and many other functions vital to life. Marginal vitamin B_{12} was found in 4 of 95 patients from this survey. Finally, carotene—the vegetable form of vitamin A—was low in 8 of 105 studied.

Because these were patients whose interest in nutrition had already led them to improve their diets or to take vitamin and mineral supplements before coming to me, they were in better shape than most people. The results would have been much worse in the general population. I can project a subclinical "walking" malnutrition for millions of Americans that will eventually result in overt illness and significant shortening of their lives.

Why Should I Worry? I Eat a Balanced Diet

For generations, medical science has acted on the presumption that all patients come before the doctor or the researcher on a nutritionally equal basis. This is one of the basic tenets of conventional medical thinking that orthomolecular experience has finally disproved. Equally illusory was the unchallenged assumption that the body somehow converts the food it eats into the nutrients it needs. This is, at best, a fuzzy concept and is the only basis for continuing to believe in the efficacy of a balanced diet. Yet we are as much individuals *under the skin* as we are *superficially;* each of us needs specific nutrients, especially micronutrients; and what we must learn is that we can't count on any magic in our digestive system to provide those nutrients.

I have made it a practice to study the individuality of people's diets wherever possible. A few years ago, I was asked to lecture to an elite group of women in San Francisco on the subject of nutrition. To involve them in my talk and to gather additional data for my work, I asked each of the 25 women to fill out a diet questionnaire beforehand, to be tabulated by computer. Of the 25, only 6 were able to maintain a diet within 80 percent or better of the RDA. I found it interesting and hopeful that the same 6 showed overt signs of good health: they were the most active and attractive women in the group. Yet the most significant finding of this small sampling was that most of the group apparently had a "well-balanced diet." All but two of them had kept their caloric intake from refined carbohydrates to less than 30 percent of their total intake—a good level. Yet further analysis showed that more than half the group were deficient in vitamins and minerals. Fat was providing 50 percent of their caloric intake—calories empty of almost all vitamins and minerals.

I see this same phenomenon of poor eating habits thinly disguised by the illusion of a balanced diet constantly in my practice. Let's look at specific cases of "micro-malnutrition."

Thirty-two-year-old Sarah L. came to me early in 1978 complaining of insomnia, fatigue, and depression. She had been experiencing these symptoms for five months and her personal physician had not been able to help her. During this time she moved into a new house and soon came down with the flu. For several months she was unable to overcome the feelings of anxiety and weakness associated with these two events. A new mother, she also felt drained by the demands of her daughter, who would wake up several times during the night to be fed. Sarah was still breast-feeding her fourteen-month-old child, well beyond the usual time of weaning. Naturally, this was depleting her, for Sarah was producing about two glasses of milk a day, an amount which was a significant drain of precious nutrients on her system. However, she considered that she was taking good nutritional care of herself, for she had been taking significant doses of vitamin C, vitamins A and D and a

Super-B complex, plus some extra iron. Even so, she was low in trace minerals and protein, due to the demands of prolonged lactation.

Her medical history showed that she had suffered a mild hypoglycemia (low blood sugar) three years before, which suggested a moderate imbalance in her hormonal regulation of sugar levels. She was slightly overweight, so she wasn't starving in the caloric sense. Her pulse rate was a bit elevated at 78, with an occasional missed beat, and her blood pressure was on the low side of normal at 100/70, but the rest of her physical examination was normal. She had a few white spots in her fingernails, which suggest mineral deficiencies, particularly zinc and manganese. Her laboratory profile showed no anemia, no disorders of the urinary tract, and generally normal levels of conventional indicators. Calcium levels and bile liver enzymes were all normal. Her copper was normal. Because she was taking vitamins, her folic acid and B_{12} were normal. Her zinc was normal (despite the "fingernail" clue) and so was her thyroid. Her triglycerides were in the low-normal range, indicating she wasn't oversensitive to carbohydrates, a good metabolic sign. Her serum magnesium level did appear to be marginal, however, which suggested to me that she might be lacking other minerals as well. In fact, I noted that the supplement she had been taking lacked minerals other than iron.

I started Sarah on an orthomolecular "insurance" program, which means that by supplementing her diet with at least the RDAs of the known vitamins and minerals, I could have reasonable assurance that she was ingesting all the nutrients in normal amounts. Three weeks later she reported she was feeling "somewhat" better. I then prescribed a diet low in carbohydrates, and supplemented it with the amino acid tryptophane and a nutrient called inositol, both of which have been reported to help sleep.

A month later, I saw her for the third time, and she told me she was feeling "much" better. When she had reduced her carbohydrates to the lowest level she had experienced ketosis, which is the point at which one's body begins to use stored fat for energy instead of using carbohydrates. This made her feel alert, but also nauseated. So I increased her carbohydrate level to about 72 grams a day, at which point she began to feel poorly again: this time she felt tired and sleepy. When we dropped her carbohydrates again to about 20 grams, just to the point at which she avoided ketosis by eating barely adequate amounts, she now felt her best—"amazingly alert, able to make decisions, not anxious."

It was obvious that the effects of carbohydrates on this woman's health were critical, so critical she could feel the results of too many carbohydrates in her loss of well-being. But now I could show her how to establish her optimum level for optimum health. This was the effect, then, that micronutrients and *dietary tuning* had in Sarah L.'s therapy. I worked with this woman from March until the first of June, and prescribed corrective diet and supplements. After only three visits she was well enough so that I didn't hear from her until the end of 1978, when I received this note in her Christmas card:

> . . . I feel absolutely fantastic, both psychologically and physically. I just wanted to let you know that I feel so good now that I tend to overdo everything. I'm not irritable, have no depression—ask my husband!—and seem to take things in stride much better than ever before in my life. Thanks so much for everything. My husband and daughter appreciate it too. It's so nice to feel like a living human being again. I'm now trying to get my mother and sister on a good nutritional regime.

Sarah's case demonstrates how dietary irregularity can lead to poor health even when all other medical indications seem normal and conventional practice fails to come to an accurate diagnosis. Or, more importantly, an effective *cure*.

These effects of dietary imbalance, when all superficial indications are that the patient is on a "good diet," occur so often in my practice that after ten years I no longer have the slightest trust in the ability of the four major food groups to produce adequate nutrition. In fact, new discoveries in orthomolecular medicine are actually showing that what is commonly thought to be a sound dietary regimen can actually make a person ill. Two examples will show you what I mean.

Recently I had a twenty-four-year-old patient referred to me from the medical ward of a nearby hospital. He maintained a high-protein, low-carbohydrate diet and had quit smoking and drinking; yet he continued to have acute symptoms of dizziness and a rapid pulse, which sometimes became a headache, tightness in the chest, hyperventilation, muscle tics, and weakness. My experience in orthomolecular medicine had taught me to relate tics and weakness to low potassium levels in the blood. Sure enough, a subsequent hair analysis showed his potassium level was very low. (Hair analysis is a new technique in which a few strands of a patient's hair can be scientifically analyzed and a measurement of trace minerals taken. I perform this test routinely on all my patients.) He promptly responded to a potassium supplement, and after I urged him to include high-potassium foods in his diet—vegetables, melons, bananas, oranges and some whole grains—he recovered fully.

Another patient, a forty-seven-year-old former intelligence agent, came to me for depression and sexual impotence. He also suffered from muscle spasms and arthritis. After having been treated for back pain and arthritis by his physicians, he eventually became overdependent on medication. His depression and alcohol excess caused him to lose his job and his wife. Then, when he lost his sexual drive, he became even more depressed and potentially suicidal. It was at this point that he was referred to me. I determined right away that he had been scrupulously avoiding animal fats because he was afraid of cholesterol and heart attacks. He had eaten no eggs or liver for years, relying heavily on skim milk and cottage cheese instead. His vegetable intake was limited to a small salad. He drank about six ounces of hard liquor every day. A hair analysis showed low magnesium, which I offset with a calcium-magnesium tablet, and I gave him folic acid to protect him against Dilantin, which had been prescribed for him as an anticonvulsant. (It is known that this drug interferes with folic acid, as well as with vitamin D and calcium.) I also put him on a diet high in liver, eggs and nuts for their high content of protein and trace minerals. Five months later he was fine, sexually active, and no longer depressed.

Here were two cases of conventional diet thinking being totally off base, to the point of actually leading to sickness. The twenty-four-year-old on the high-protein, low-carbohydrate diet who didn't smoke or drink had a potassium deficiency that affected his life dramatically. The intelligence agent who was afraid of heart attacks and so avoided eggs and liver was low in magnesium, folic acid and the micronutrients. While these cases were medically a bit more complex than I present them here, they serve to show that the conventional view of the "well-balanced diet" is hopelessly inadequate.

A Funny Thing Happened to Your Dinner on the Way to the Table

There is no doubt in my mind that American food technology is largely responsible for the difficulty of getting a diet sufficient for optimum health in this country. For reasons of economics and distribution, the food industry has processed virtually all the natural nutrients out of the everyday food we eat. Anyone who thinks differently, including physicians and traditional dietitians, is either nutritionally naive or ignorant of the chemical makeup of the food he puts in his mouth. These are strong statements. Let's examine them in detail.

Since the technology of canning foods and milling grains was developed in the mid-19th century, the trend has been for *processed* foods—nutritionally altered foods—to make up an increasingly greater part of the American daily diet. We are learning, unfortunately, that the more processed foods we eat, the fewer nutrients we receive. It's as simple as that.

In 1940, processed foods represented only 10 percent of the American diet, whereas in 1970 they made up about 50 percent; now, merely a decade later, they comprise about 60 percent. The trend is accelerating. This is significant because the average American is severely limited by reasons of budget and convenience to processed foods. The results are increasing dietary shortages and "micro-malnutrition." Dr. Roger Williams, discoverer of the vitamin pantothenic acid and Professor of Chemistry Emeritus of the University of Texas at Austin, stated the case directly in an article for food chemists in the journal *American Laboratory:* "How do people get perfect nutrition—every item in just the right amount? The answer is, 'They don't.'"

There used to be a real balanced diet. It was real for our grandparents, whose foods were mainly unprocessed. Today, though, as Dr. Williams put it, "A perfect food environment is as rare as a perfect climatic environment." We have no way of knowing where our food originated and how much has been done to it from farm to dinner table.

What was once the "staff of life" no longer supports life. An experiment by Dr. Williams showed that rats fed only white-flour bread died within six weeks, while a comparison group of rats fed only whole-wheat bread thrived indefinitely. Rats aren't human beings, and human beings don't try to survive on bread alone, but the point is obvious.

Dr. Edith Weir, of the United States Department of Agriculture (USDA), reported in 1971 that if we all ate according to the recommended RDA levels, about 300,000 deaths a year from heart disease and stroke and 150,000 deaths from cancer could be prevented. Today the statistics would be even worse. This constitutes sufficient evidence that we're not getting even the minimal RDA level of nutrition from our supposed balance of foods.

Richard A. Passwater, a pioneering biochemist and author of *Supernutrition for Healthy Hearts,* believes that our diets are so lacking in essential nutrients that if we were to increase our intake of vitamins and minerals, heart disease would be reduced by 60–80 percent; cancer would be reduced by 30–40 percent; "damage" to the lungs would be reduced by 95 percent; the cure rate for schizophrenia would increase 500 percent; and that arthritis and similar crippling diseases would drop 40 percent.

Dr. Jean Mayer, former Presidential Nutrition Advisor and Chairman of the 1969 White House Conference on Food, Nutrition and Health, reported that since 1950 the life expectancy for adult American males is shorter than that of almost 30 other nations and that "malnutrition . . . contributes to the alarming health situation in the United States today."

These figures all underscore an attitude that I consider to be equivalent to a death sentence: "I can get all the vitamins and minerals I need from a well-balanced diet." The problem is that "balance" is no substitute for nutrients, and nutrients from food are becoming more and more difficult to get.

On its way from the "garden to the gullet," as Dr. Emanuel Cheraskin, of the University of Alabama School of Medicine, puts it, the food on your table has had 50 percent of its nutrients removed. Dr. Cheraskin has been a leader in nutritional research for the past 30 years. A study by Cheraskin and his colleague, W. M. Ringsdorf, M.D., showed how a "typical" dinner plate of pork chops, potato, and vegetable has been nutritionally mugged on its way to your digestive system.

To begin with, food derives its nutritional strength from the soil it's grown in. But the mineral content of much of the nation's arable soil has been vastly reduced over the years by various factors, chief among which has been the continuous poisoning of the land by insecticides and chemicals. When crops are ready for harvesting, we may conservatively say that about 10 percent of their nutritional value has been lost. The calories remain but the micronutrients—numerous vitamins and minerals —are depleted. The nutritional losses from modern methods of feeding livestock and poultry are even greater.

During the time it takes to transport them to the store, fruits and vegetables have lost perhaps another 10 percent of their micronutrient value. One study, in fact, showed that a carrot eaten by an American has fewer nutrients than a carrot eaten by his Mexican counterpart, simply because in Mexico—usually considered an underdeveloped and agriculturally poor nation—the carrot was probably grown less than a mile from his home. The American's carrot was probably grown hundreds of miles away; this leaves you now with 80 percent.

What about the lengthy storage in the grocery store? This can remove at least another 10 percent, especially from meats and vegetables, so your meal now has only 70 percent of its starting nutritional value.

Americans eat an enormous amount of foods that have been, at one time or another, frozen. Meat is kept frozen in your freezer until you decide to eat it; some vegetables and fruit are chilled or frozen in railroad cars or trucks on their way to your supermarket. The logistics of transporting and preserving food in transport also results in a nutritional loss not even calculated here: most produce is picked or harvested green, before it has a chance to reach its full nutritional value. Since food loses 5 percent to 10 percent of its nutrients in the defrosting process, let's say conservatively that you now have 65 percent of the original food values on your plate.

Washing food takes away many valuable minerals and vitamins, which are most abundant on the skins and outer layers of fruits and vegetables. This you could control, but usually you don't even *get* the outer layers: most produce men strip the dark, "imperfect" leaves off the vegetables before they put them out. Vitamins and minerals carpet the floor of the produce room. Let's estimate another 5 percent loss, leaving us with 60 percent of the original micronutrients.

Now we must consider the way we usually prepare the food after it comes home. Boiling, baking, and overcooking food greatly reduce nutritional value. As much as 50 percent of the nutrients in vegetables are removed by the standard method of cooking, say, spinach and broccoli, which is usually to boil them to death. Conservatively, you have burned out of your well-done meat and boiled out of your overcooked vegetables about 20 percent of their original nutrients. Again, you can control this to some extent—but most of us don't. We now have on our plates 40 percent of the micronutritional value of the food as it was grown or raised.

Other things to consider: insecticides on your fruit; preservatives (to keep that slice of bread "fresh"); additives (to make those beets redder); processing (for that cheese spread); sweeteners (like the sugar added to your catsup). The chemical reaction of these agents with the nutrients in your food can often render vitamins and minerals inactive, essentially inert; the food might as well not have any nutrients at all. We shall investigate the poisonous effects of these chemicals on your body in another chapter. Conservatively, we can say that they can reduce food values by half, leaving only 20 percent of the original nutrients on your table.

Admittedly, this demonstration can vary dramatically with particular foods and with the family preparing them. Many people cultivate a garden of some sort and eat vegetables fresh from their own backyard several times a week during the summer. Many poeple are also conscious of their diets and shun foods that they know to be processed, shipped or frozen. Nevertheless, the majority of Americans today have an exaggerated idea of food values and think that "getting all the vitamins and minerals they need" simply means a visit to the supermarket. The Cheraskin study shows that to get the nutrients your grandparents had you would have to eat three or four times the amount of food they did, if supermarket food is your only source of nutrition.

Fresh, Frozen, or Canned? That Is the Question

What specific nutrients are lost in processing and refining? Let's look at some scientifically derived figures to substantiate our theoretical approximations. Henry A. Schroeder, M.D., writing in the *American Journal of Clinical Nutrition,* recently reported the results of extensive laboratory analysis of many foods for their concentrations of essential trace minerals and vitamin B_6 and pantothenic acid. More than 700 foods and edible products were analyzed, including 83 varieties of baby foods. Comparisons were made of 58 canned foods and 32 frozen foods with their raw counterparts, including seafoods, meats, dairy products, and vegetables.

The results clearly corroborate the Cheraskin study. Here are some samples:

Seafoods: The B_6 content in raw herring was 3.70 micrograms per gram and in frozen herring 3.20, while in canned herring it was 1.60. The B_6 content (micrograms per gram) in raw mackerel was 6.60, frozen was 4.10, and canned was 2.80.

The pantothenic acid in herring went from 9.70 raw to 7.00 canned. It went from 8.50 to 5.00 in mackerel.

Meats: The B_6 content of chicken went from 6.83 fresh to 3.00 canned, and pork went from 4.50 to 2.70.

Vegetables: The B_6 content of carrots went from 1.50 micrograms fresh to 0.30 canned; in potatoes from 2.50 to 1.02; in peas from 1.60 to 0.50.

In terms of *average loss percentage,* the fish products lost 17.3 percent when frozen and 48.9 percent when canned. The root vegetables (carrots and potatoes) lost 63.1 percent when canned. The legume vegetables (peas, beans) lost 55.6 percent when frozen and 77.4 percent when canned.

I have no precise figures for depletion due to poor soil and washing and cooking, but, of course, even fresh produce suffers from this nutritional loss.

Dr. Schroeder concludes on a hopeful note: "Foods with an excess of micronutrients, i.e., vitamins and minerals, are needed to compensate for foods with less than adequate amounts in order that the total intake may supply the body's requirements. It is apparent that raw foods supply adequate amounts of all the micronutrients here considered." Schroeder says that persons subsisting on refined, processed and canned foods will *not* be provided with adequate amounts. Intakes may be seriously marginal for those on reducing diets and for older persons whose caloric intakes may be limited because of relative inactivity.

Strong stuff. Not only is the "balanced diet" a thing of the past for most Americans, but *nonfoods* have infiltrated every meal: colas, pastries, candy, condiments, and so forth. Dr. George Briggs, professor of nutrition at the University of California at Berkeley, told a health seminar recently that 50 percent of the American diet is composed of nonessential foods, and that when we dilute our diets as much as 25 percent we "begin to run into health problems." People who ignore the threat of micro-malnutrition "are likely to suffer the consequences of disease unless they remedy their eating habits," and he goes on to say, "It [disease] often shows up 15 or 20 years later in the form of softening of the bones, diabetes, heart disease, or other nutrition-related disease."

Aside from the hazards of processed foods and nonfoods, there are two other sources of "empty calories" to keep in mind:

1. The fat intake in the American diet accounts for 45 percent of food calories.
2. The refined sugar intake alone, not counting alcoholic beverages and other refined carbohydrates, averages 120 grams per day, which is almost 500 calories, or 25 percent of the calories ingested by most sedentary adults.

"Empty-calorie" foods obviously do not provide their share of vitamins and minerals. With fats and sugars making up 70 percent of the average American diet, where are the nutrients coming from? The other 30 percent is the difference between life and death, sickness and health.

It is this vital 30 percent that has to run the gauntlet of freezing, canning, milling, washing and cooking.

Who Is the Real Food Faddist: Betty Crocker or Adelle Davis?

If you were to ask the president of the American Medical Association, "Doctor, is the American diet adequate?" the reply would be "yes." The medical profession closed the book on nutrition in the 1940s when it seemed that all the essential nutrients had been discovered. Enrichment of flour, fortification of milk, and teaching children about the four basic food groups were believed to be sufficient to end malnutrition.

For some 40 years we have had "enriched flour." Enriched! They took out 20 essential nutrients in the process of refining the flour, and then put back 4, and they call it "enriched." It has been argued that white flour is at least better than none, but second-rate food tends to drive out the best. So I'm not so sure. The price we're paying is an epidemic of cancer, heart disease, arthritis, diabetes, and a host of other maladies. But I also believe that the lessons we have learned from the disaster of overrefined foods are beginning to swing the balance the other way. We are at the frontier of a revolution that will restore nutrition to a central role in medicine.

It is difficult to imagine now, but politics played a leading role in supposedly scientific decisions in the medical world some years ago. In 1939 the entire field of nutrition was essentially banished from medical teaching and practice. In a series of political actions the pro-nutritionists were battered down in the pages of scientific journals and even investigated by government agencies. Popular writers like Adelle Davis were ridiculed for their "food faddism." Only a handful persisted to point the way for latter-day orthomolecular physicians and psychiatrists (although the word "orthomolecular" wasn't coined until later) to begin investigating for themselves the value of micronutrients in medical work.

When my work was first written up in *Prevention* magazine some years ago, it was pointed out that I was among the first to do hair analysis to determine mineral levels. I was the first to use pubic hair in this procedure because it's contaminated by air exposure less often, and rarely contaminated by shampoos, sprays, dyes, etc. I was the first to discover that the skin flush reaction to the B vitamin niacin is blocked by aspirin and thus reflects prostaglandin activity. (Prostaglandins are a newly discovered class of hormones.) And I was the first to find that manganese is a powerful factor in protecting the nerve cells against bad effects of some tranquilizers.

I point out this background because in what I have to say about diet and disease throughout the rest of this book I want you to know the source of my opinions. I am going to show how my 10 years of ortho-molecular work (coming after almost 20 years of conventional prac-tice) have convinced me that traditional medical practice has ignored one of the pillars of medicine: diet. Instead we've relied only on the other three: drugs, surgery, and psychotherapy. While most doctors are expert at surgery and pharmacology and treasure the "art of medicine," few have even tried diet. Those of us who have tried it find it works. It's that simple.

Health foods—nine-grain bread, raw vegetables, and nuts, for exam-ple—are called faddist. But the true fad is the processed diet. *It* is the departure from nature. Health foods manufacturers are not allowed to make claims, while drug manufacturers bombard physicians in practi-cally every medical journal with expensive four-color advertisements. The health food industry and the growing society of orthomolecular medical practitioners are the ones who advocate a return to the basics of nature—whole foods—containing the molecules of nutrients which are essential to develop and sustain life.

The danger in the processed diet, the mythical "balanced diet" of America today, is the lack of such molecules. If our diet withholds *any* of the vital nutrients from our bodies, it leaves us somewhat defenseless. We must constantly replenish the molecules which support the functions of the body—growth, resistance to disease, maintenance of chemical balance. This is the basis of orthomolecular medicine, or orthomedicine for short.

Orthomedicine depends to some extent on supplementing your avail-able food with a high-potency vitamin and mineral tablet. It should be one that provides near-RDA levels of vitamins, minerals, and perhaps small amounts of some amino acids. The radiant good health of patients tells me that this advice alone—the daily use of a supplement—will re-duce the threat of the "killer diseases" for anyone who gives it a try. For the basic killer is malnutrition that never shows itself until it's too late, when we call it heart disease or diabetes or cancer.

The Nutrition Prescription for Subclinical Malnutrition

- Think first in terms of raw foods
- Increase your vegetable intake in general
- Make a point to get at least two servings of "whole" foods a day—those foods that have not been altered from their natural form
- Where cooking is absolutely necessary, don't overcook and do use any liquids resulting from cooking in soups or gravies
- Avoid white bread and add grains—whole-grain breads, wheat cereals, oatmeal, brown rice—to your diet at least once a day
- Make it a habit to take a multi-vitamin/mineral supplement each morning

3

The Malnutrition of Obesity

I first became interested in obesity when a relative of mine died as a result of a "successful" reducing diet. She had retained the vitality and grace that had won her a lifetime of admiration as a great beauty and dedicated teacher until she was sixty-three. At that age, she had become somewhat overweight and with characteristic discipline had cut her food intake drastically. Her reduced diet, unfortunately, did not include vitamin supplements. Following her doctor's orders she managed to lose 35 pounds, and it resulted in her death.

Does one drop dead of malnutrition? Yes! Here's how it happens. Strictly speaking, the proximate cause of my relative's death was a heart attack, and that was the official explanation. She had never been seriously ill, was moderate in her habits, and could boast a hereditary "edge": her mother had lived to the age of ninety-seven. I consider her a victim of nutritional and metabolic ignorance that can kill one in gaining weight or in losing weight—especially the latter in our fashion-conscious, nutrition-naive society.

The heart attack has become a facile villain. Consider another case.

A few months after this woman's death, I lost a good friend—forty years of age, the same story. He had just lost 30 pounds under doctor's orders. Nicely trimmed down, he went out for a game of basketball with his son. After a fast-paced hour he collapsed with a fatal heart stoppage.

How naive it is for anyone, let alone a physician, to think that a restricted diet, sufficiently reduced in calories to accomplish a major weight loss, would not also be dangerously low in vital nutrients. Not just desirable nutrients, but *vital* ones. A shortage of nutrients, such as occurs in an improperly managed weight loss diet, can aggravate preexisting heart disease or possibly *cause* heart stoppage and death. Neither of the two people who were dear to me had had preexisting heart disease. But a prolonged dietary deficiency can be the real villain in a case of "heart attack."

Fat and Starving

That one can be overweight, even obese, but still dangerously undernourished is also a difficult concept to grasp. The majority of people have been so ill informed by the press, by word-of-mouth misinformation, and by mythology that we have begun to relate overweight with overabundance. We go on believing, as a supposedly overfed nation, that *reducing* our intake of food doesn't seriously reduce our vital nutrient intake.

The rule that makes most sense to me is this: when it comes to nutrients, better too much than too little. Weight loss always requires a state of temporary undernutrition. To put it bluntly, weight loss means some degree of starvation. If it were not so, there could be no weight loss. A *properly managed* program means only one thing: to accomplish the weight loss with a *minimum* of starvation. Cut down on calories but don't cut down on vital nutrients. *Optimizing* your personal, individual diet is the aim of "orthomedical" weight control—not merely to maintain weight at some arbitrary level but to achieve optimum health. How an "ortho" program works in practice is the subject of Chapter 15.

Optimum weight is only one sign of optimum health. *Overweight is always a sign of impaired health.* Obesity invites a Pandora's box of complications and associated diseases. An excessive accumulation of fat in the body overworks the heart, causes shortness of breath, increases blood pressure, and leads to diabetes, chronic back and joint pains, varicose veins, edema (swelling), and susceptibility to infectious diseases. It goes without saying that obesity poses psychological problems as well: it represents an overall immobility that reduces one's ability to enjoy life.

I define overweight and obesity—as the actuaries do—in percentages. You are "overweight" if you are between 10 and 20 percent more than an optimum weight for your age and height and "obese" if you are more than 20 percent overweight. Hence, if you are a 6-foot male of moderate build and your desirable weight is said to be 180 pounds by the standard charts, you're overweight up to 216 pounds and obese if you weigh even more. The point at which you want to start doing something about it is, of course, up to you.

Obesity is so commonplace that people may believe the condition is normal. One study of the records of 26 life insurance companies found that weights of both men and women were, on the average, 15 to 25 pounds too high, and that 30 percent of the men and 40 percent of the women over the age of forty were obese. At a figure of 40 percent, it's easy for people to believe it's a normal condition.

One such case came to my attention not long ago. Shirley was 5 feet 6 inches tall, the 190-pound divorced mother of two teenage daughters. Always a good cook, she prided herself too much on her delicacies, even after she began to lose the battle of the bulge. Intermittent fad diets took their toll. She repeatedly lost and regained 30 pounds until finally she developed persistent headache and stomach pain as well as stretch marks over her otherwise unblemished skin.

X-ray examination of her stomach revealed lax ligaments in the diaphragm, permitting her stomach to herniate into her chest—a hiatus hernia. This was the cause of her persistent heartburn, for stomach juices could flow back into the lower esophagus. Whenever she ate, particularly proteins and fats, she would suffer severely as the acid juices of the stomach increased and worked their way onto the inflamed tissues of the esophagus. Antacids only made her feel worse and finally she was forced by pain to limit her diet to milk, yogurt, fish, whole-wheat cereal, and cooked vegetables. No medication seemed to help despite the attention of many physicians in the two years before she consulted me. Because she was already taking vitamin supplements before she came to me, her laboratory findings were initially normal. However, she almost fainted during the glucose tolerance test, despite the fact that her blood sugar values never went below 52 milligrams per 100 milliliters. This is usually considered within normal limits but for her it was too low. She had to bundle up because of chills for the last two hours of the test.

Vitamin therapy did not seem to help her, possibly because stomach pain caused her to be erratic in her diet and vitamin intake. An attempt to lower her carbohydrate intake failed because she couldn't tolerate much protein or fat and felt weak and shaky on a low-carbohydrate diet. Her condition, which had been worsening before consulting me, continued to deteriorate. Soon she could eat only milk, yams and vege-table soup.

In desperation I prescribed a total fast in order to rest the inflamed tissues. Within three days she was improved and after three weeks of ingesting only water she was symptom-free. In this time she lost only 8 pounds, however, indicating that she must have retained at least 10 pounds of fluid in her tissues. Otherwise, weight could have been ex-pected to drop by twice that amount or more. That would be more than a gallon of water retention, not a sign of good health. When she re-sumed eating, her symptoms recurred at once. I referred her to a com-petent and conscientious gastroenterologist, who found reflux esopha-gitis by examining her with fiberoptic light and viewing the tube in her esophagus and stomach. He rated her disorder as "mild." Since antacids and antispasmodics didn't help her, nor did the psyllium seed bulk agent that he prescribed, she returned to me a month later, as desperate as ever. Now I recommended zucchini broth, a good nutrient without digestive problems, favored by the late Dr. Hans Bieler, a pioneer in nu-tritional medicine. This was helpful, but she was unable to branch out into a full diet: the broth and milk were her staples. After a few months, she suddenly developed a papular rash (small, inflamed bumps or pim-ples) over most of her body as well as mild but distinct inflammation and scaling of her eyelids. Water retention was sufficient to produce ex-cessive swelling of her ankles. Her liver was slightly tender and she was exhausted.

These symptoms indicated malnutrition, so I referred her again to the gastroenterologist in hopes that he might hospitalize her and provide in-travenous feeding or help her to obtain a predigested elemental diet. I felt she had to take a load off her digestive system, but this was not my specialty. He did not feel that this was indicated, however, despite the fact that the ingestion of even a glass of water now caused bloating, and eating anything was followed by a choking sensation from her inflamed esophagus. He did try the newly available histamine blocking agent, Cimetidine, but it proved ineffective.

Since she was a Medicaid patient, I did not have as free a hand in treating her with certain medications or elemental diet products because they were not on the approved list. I was so concerned that she was going downhill that after the gastroenterologist finally diagnosed her as "hysterical," I referred her to a general practitioner. This doctor did admit her to his hospital because of her distress, but let her go within a few days because he couldn't satisfy himself that she had any disease other than psychophysiological disorder, i.e., "nervous stomach."

Despite my pleas to attend to her malnutrition, these fine and concerned physicians were put off by her obesity. She still weighed about 187 pounds, due mostly to the intake of milk, which is high in calories (about 600 per quart). Nevertheless, I knew that the skin changes, hair loss, and persistent esophageal pain indicated inability to heal and had to be due to malnutrition.

The irony of it all was that the laboratory tests I had recommended to the doctor while she was in the hospital for a few days now came to me after she had been discharged from the hospital. Several nutrients were deficient: magnesium, zinc, and vitamin A. How was she to heal when deficient in vitamin A and zinc, both of which are necessary for the manufacture of new tissues by our body's cells?

In response to these findings, I started injecting vitamins, as well as prescribing applications of safflower oil to the skin. (It is known that the essential fatty acids in safflower oil can be absorbed directly into the body that way.) In ten days her heartburn cleared up for the first time in a year, the first time since the total fast. The use of a histamine blocking agent, to reduce stomach acidity, and a two-week partial fast, relying on fruit and vegetable juices, also helped. With the fast her skin rash and eyelids cleared up, and we now realized that she must have had a milk allergy. This process of elimination is a reliable way to determine allergies. By pursuing this treatment and eliminating dairy products from her diet, not only did she clear her skin but she also healed her stomach.

This case, although concerned with clinical medicine and allergies, clearly shows that an overweight person, even one who takes some nutritional supplements, can be dangerously lacking in essential nutrients. It also shows how conventional medicine can be so intent upon finding a standard medical diagnosis that it ignores the possibility of nutritional disturbance. Orthomolecular medicine uncovered her deficiencies, corrected them, and in the process diagnosed her allergy to milk products. Otherwise, she might have continued to be regarded as "hysterical."

The most important point is that she was *fat and starving!* Experienced medical specialists were unable to appreciate this even when the laboratory tests indicated malnutrition. Many of the patients who consult with me for weight problems have similar nutrient deficiencies. They are *overweight and undernourished*.

One of the greatest, yet least understood dangers of obesity is the yo-yo syndrome: recurrent nutrient deficiences induced by repeated efforts at weight reduction through dieting—and repeated failures. I am distressed when I examine my overweight patients and find their bodies damaged, not from obesity but from self-induced starvation. Sagging skin and telltale stretch marks need not occur; they are probably caused by deficiency of protein or certain trace elements, particularly zinc or copper, or in some cases by lack of vitamin C, which is also essential in maintenance of connective tissues. It is unpleasant to have to tell a young person, especially an attractive woman, that her thighs, abdomen and breasts will always bear testimony to a time of undernutrition.

So, overweight has its dangers: in addition to the danger of recurrent malnutrition of the yo-yo syndrome and the danger of a serious metabolic imbalance—and even death due to crash dieting—there are the well-known morbidities associated with obesity itself. If you are obese, the risk of sudden death from all causes is three and a half times greater than at your optimal weight, and death from coronary heart disease and diabetes is almost twice as likely.

Why We Go to Fat

Why then does anyone become overweight? If it has so many disadvantages, why should anyone let it happen? The obvious answer to this important question is: people get fat because they eat too much. But it isn't so simple. Careful studies of overweight humans have shown without a doubt that some people remain overweight while eating less than normal. As little as 800 calories per day has been known to maintain weight in some cases. How can this be?

Without going into too much detail, let's recall that food energy is measured in calories. The calories in food are converted into chemical energy, heat, and movement in the body. If the amount of energy intake exceeds energy use, the excess energy is stored as fat tissue. If the energy use of the body cells is reduced, even a relatively small intake of calories may maintain or even cause a gain in weight. Now, it just so happens that when one is undernourished, the control mechanisms of the body reduce energy use within a very few weeks, in most people. This is because of reduction in thyroid activity, which normally controls the energy consumption of the body's cells. Low thyroid means that the physical movement and pulse rate are lower than when the thyroid is activated. So, it's not surprising to find that actual studies of obese people have revealed a significant decrease in physical movement and activity.

It sounds as if it would be simple to solve the problem of obesity by simply administering thyroid supplements, doesn't it? Well, this has been done and it sometimes helps. However, often it does not. The reason for this is that *under*nutrition also reduces the body's output of another class of hormones called catecholamines. These are similar to adrenaline, the "flight or fight" hormone. It is the diminished supply of both catecholamines and adrenaline that accounts for the fact that in fasting most people feel cold but also calmer and less aggressive.

An additional reason why starving people tend to be less active than the well-fed is that, when one is starving, the fat deposits are being burned. This produces another chemical substance, ketones (chemical fragments of fats), which have a tranquilizing action of their own.

Is it possible to administer a catecholamine drug to fight obesity? The answer is "yes"! And the drug is called amphetamine or "speed." But since amphetamines can be dangerous, they have recently been made illegal as a treatment for obesity, despite the fact that for many years a combination of thyroid hormone and amphetamine was successfully used by physicians. In short-term treatment it was not dangerous; however, long-term exposure may cause addiction, paranoia, and some brain damage.

Many Ways to Gain, Few to Lose

If it sounds easier to gain weight than to lose, you are right. This is especially so if you have a hereditary tendency toward obesity. There is no doubt that heredity does contribute to body build. Ease of weight gain is certainly characteristic of some families. This has been studied from many points of view in mice that have been bred specially for obesity. In such mice, the offspring will almost always become obese. One particularly intriguing observation in the obese strain of mice is that mild stress increases obesity. By merely pinching their tails a few times a day, one can provoke weight gains. Hereditarily lean mice are not so affected by stress. If similar mechanisms apply in humans, hereditarily obese types will gain weight under stress, while hereditarily lean types may lose weight.

A winner of the Nobel Prize, Rosalyn Yalow, discovered that a hormone, cholecystokinin, which is known to block appetite and induce satiety when introduced into the brain of mammals is deficient in hereditarily obese mice. Furthermore, psychologists at Temple and Tufts universities and other investigators at the National Institutes of Health have demonstrated an increase in the hormone beta endorphin in the pituitary glands of obese mice and rats. This hormone, which is known to mimic the effects of opiates, was present at double the concentration in the pituitary glands of obese animals as compared to normal. When a drug to block the formation of opiates was administered to these animals, it stopped their overeating. Yet the same dose in lean mice was of no effect; it did not decrease their normal eating.

Does increasing the cholecystokinin in humans curtail appetite? This has, indeed, been demonstrated. But how can this be accomplished? Nature has provided a simple answer. Cholecystokinin is produced by cells of the small intestine. When fat, from a fatty meal, reaches the intestine it stimulates release of cholecystokinin, which then causes the gallbladder to contract, thus mobilizing the bile to ensure proper digestion of the fat. It also acts on the brain, where we now know it has an important role in controlling appetite. The presence of fat in the meal is well known to appease appetite. This may account for the fact that a high-fat diet has been shown to cause a reduction in caloric intake! It is on this basis that the high-fat, low-carbohydrate Atkins diet may actually work for some people.

On the other hand, there are also substances produced from proteins and carbohydrates that turn off hunger, though not so rapidly or clearly as does fat. It is believed that these substances are produced in the liver, and some speculation has it that the loss of appetite in liver disease states, particularly hepatitis and cancer, is somehow related to the change in liver production of these substances.

Why We Eat—Why When We Eat Is Important

Our understanding of how our bodies control their weight is turning out to be rather more complicated than was expected when the "appestat" theory of hunger was introduced 30 years ago. At that time it was believed that there were glucoreceptors, sugar-sensitive cells, in the hypothalamus of the brain, an almond-sized area adjacent to the pituitary gland. When the sugar level went down, the appetite was believed to go up and vice versa. (The appestat tells you when you are hungry and turns on your appetite.)

On the basis of that theory, some practitioners recommended that eating sugar is the quickest and best way to turn off hunger. That was before it was appreciated that sugar, particularly sucrose (table sugar), strongly stimulates insulin and thus causes a rebound low-blood-sugar effect. Sugar stimulates hunger from one to three hours after eating, thus provoking overeating and overweight.

While the mechanisms are still under study, it does appear that the act of eating expresses a dynamic interaction between hunger cells located in the outer part of the hypothalamus (lateral nuclei) and satiety cells located in the inner part (ventral-medial nuclei). The activation level of this appestat is affected by numerous physiochemical and emotional factors.

Frequency of meals is often very important in weight control. Dr. Paul Fabry, of the Institute for Clinical and Experimental Medicine in Prague, found that eating a few large meals promoted the accumulation of fat and weight gain more than eating several smaller meals adding up to the same calories. He found, too, that in older people, fewer large meals promoted increased cholesterol and higher blood sugar levels than the smaller meal regimen. (His finding was that 58.2 percent of those on three meals a day were overweight, while only 28.8 percent of those on five small meals or more per day were overweight.)

Furthermore, the shift from nibbling to eating large meals (gorging) leads to changes in the body chemistry that favor the buildup of fat. Dr. Clarence Cohn fed one group of rats by stomach tube twice a day and compared their weight to a second group that nibbled freely the same amount of food. After 41 days the force-fed rats all had more body fat. Dr. Ernest Leveille repeated the study without force-feeding, instead merely limiting the time during which food was available. In a few weeks, the meal-fed rats had consumed 15 percent fewer calories than the nibbling group, yet they had gained the same amount of weight. Leveille reports that when nibbling rats are switched to meal-eating, the maximum rate of fat synthesis is attained within nine days; the adipose tissue increases severalfold its ability to convert glucose to fat. However, when meal-fed rats are returned to nibbling, it takes six weeks to readapt, i.e., to lose this increased ability to store fat.

Leveille concluded that obesity is the result of eating habits, a behavioral rather than a metabolic fault. The fault is the habit of eating meals at widely separated periods each day.

What We Can Learn from the Fads

As it stands now, the large number of factors that influence personality, appetite, body chemistry and activity, which together determine whether we are fat or lean, are so complex that successful treatment of obesity must be determined by your own makeup. The fact that there have been so many ingenious—and sometimes ridiculous—fad diets is the best evidence of the complex nature of the problem. For example, why was the liquid protein "Last Chance diet" so popular? It is actually based upon scientific principles derived from research at Harvard and the University of Texas. The researchers were able to provide all of the essential nutrients in their method. Their diet was called a "protein-sparing modified fast" in the scientific journals, because, by providing sufficient protein, along with essential fatty acids and micronutrients, the amount of protein nitrogen lost in the urine was less than the amount in the food ingested. In other words, the body chemical metabolism was so efficient that it could conserve its own protein. Since protein is the essential stuff of which the body is made, this protected the body from deteriorating during the weight reduction period. Because of the remarkable success of the diet in the setting of the university metabolic ward, it was rushed into general use before all of the wrinkles had been ironed out. Resistant cases were able to lose weight comfortably. The method worked even with retarded children who were grossly overweight.

Nevertheless, I am sure that you would not want to try this diet on yourself. In May, 1978, the FDA issued a bulletin based on 165 complaints and reports of injuries and more than 40 adverse reports by physicians on behalf of their patients who had tried one liquid protein diet. The FDA projected an annual rate of 59 deaths due to sudden cardiac death without underlying heart disease per 100,000 women aged twenty-five to forty-four, a 30-fold increase over the expected 2 deaths per 100,000 in this age group.

Of the three cases reported in the *New England Journal of Medicine*, two died after five months on liquid protein and weight losses of 40 to 85 pounds. Minor deficiencies of potassium and magnesium were found, not enough to account for the electrical disorders of the heart that proved fatal. The medical profession was particularly alarmed by these fatalities because many of the patients were actually under medical supervision and taking vitamin and potassium supplements. If not for this, even more injuries would have resulted, for the liquid protein diet is low in calcium, magnesium, potassium, and copper. Dr. Leslie Klevay has calculated that four months on the liquid protein diet, which contains almost no copper whatsoever, would use up the body stores of copper. Inflammation of the heart and heart stoppage is typical in laboratory animals with low copper. Serious deficiency of magnesium and potassium can have the same consequences.

Although they are not part of my practice, for anyone who does follow a liquid protein diet I would advise supplementing the protein with the missing amino acids as well as the missing minerals. Even with that, it should not be continued over three months at a time but should be interrupted frequently by a period of nutritious eating to be sure that no vital nutrient is depleted.

When the Last Chance diet turned into exactly that for those who died as a result, almost everyone was scared away from all special diets for weight loss. Instead the "balanced" diet returned to popularity as people recoiled in fear from anything that seemed like a fad diet. Most recently the Scarsdale diet has gained popularity. It assigns a daily menu plan for weight loss that is spelled out day by day for two weeks. It is popular because it works and because it is so precise. There are no decisions to make, thus it resolves the fear and confusion left by the liquid protein diet. But the Scarsdale diet is not completely safe either and is specifically limited to three weeks. It is obviously deficient in essential fatty acids because the use of vegetable oil or fat is prohibited in the instructions. The only fat in the diet is saturated animal fat, contained in meat, cheese and eggs. Moreover, the diet does not insist on whole-grain bread, which would provide trace minerals, nor does it provide nuts or beans or other nutrient-rich foods. Weight loss will occur in the first few weeks, but if the diet is followed beyond that time, most people will start to feel tired or else they will develop hunger cravings that will interrupt the diet. This diet should be seen as a two-stage procedure, with modifications necessary for long-term use.

At times of distrust of diet fads, a majority of people rely on their own common sense to plan a "balanced" weight loss diet. This usually means reducing portions and cutting out sweets entirely. Unfortunately, with the reduced amount of food eaten it is likely that even a "common sense" diet will be lacking in nutrients. The result can be quite frightening.

Anne came to see me at the urging of her friend, who became alarmed when she fainted at work. A strikingly beautiful woman, she was also ambitious and very strong-willed. She had succumbed to the desire for an "ideal" figure and thus set about to restrict her food intake for prolonged periods to keep herself at 110 pounds, which she felt was best for her height of 5 feet 6 inches. It was my impression that she could carry 10 extra pounds with greater health and therefore more appeal. The day that she fainted she had stood behind a store counter all day without eating. When she did eat, her diet was restricted to fish, meat and vegetables, with no dairy, egg, grains, nuts or fruit, which she considered "fattening."

My physical examination showed Anne to be normal except for low blood pressure, only 80/45 (normal range 110 to 130 over 60 to 80). But the laboratory reports were more revealing. She was mildly anemic, her red cell count reduced to 3.84 million (normal 4.2 million) and her hemoglobin was only 11.4 grams (normal 12 to 14 grams). Serum magnesium was only 1.4 milligrams per deciliter (normal 1.8 to 2.5). Serum iron was low.

I instructed her in the use of supplements and encouraged her to improve her diet, as described in Chapter 15. She experienced an immediate 4-pound weight gain and signs of fluid retention. She worked it off in her typical fashion, taking a 2-mile swim. She said she felt "enormous" at 115 pounds and there was no persuading her to enjoy a more natural weight. Therefore, I concentrated on helping her to get all the essential nutrients she needed. She looked and felt better within a few weeks and has maintained her improvement in well-being even though she still weighs only 110 pounds.

Others among my patients have tried to accomplish weight loss by simply reducing their portions of all foods. Unfortunately, this induces undersupply of several micronutrients, not just calories, and causes irresistible cravings that usually culminate in a food binge. Food binges may bring momentary relief from the hunger of dieting but the afterpangs of guilt, resentment, and grief are painful indeed. It is so demoralizing to be unable to keep control of one's own body that many obese people refuse to get on a scale. Words like "diet" and "calories" become unpleasant and are avoided. Eventually, many obese people ignore logical connections between food and feelings. Fat people often eat automatically; they don't even know they are eating. At that point, the need for help is so great that anything that sounds simple and promises quick results is likely to be irresistible.

Dangers and Rewards of Fasting

Fasting as a means of weight loss is one fad that has been carefully studied. In the *Archives of Internal Medicine,* 1977, Drs. Daisie Johnson and Ernst Drenick reported that total fasting was well tolerated as a means of weight loss for the morbidly obese. However, most of their 207 subjects regained the weight they lost while fasting. At the start, the average weight of these patients was 310 pounds. Half of them fasted for two months and lost an average of 66 pounds; others went on to lose even more weight. After three years, however, 50 percent of the patients had regained their original weight and when they were contacted nine years later fewer than 10 percent had maintained any weight loss whatsoever. A repeat fast was attempted by 25 of these patients, but this also failed to achieve lasting benefits.

I must issue this warning: *Prolonged fasting should be carefully observed* and, as a rule, be undertaken with hospital supervision, as it can be extremely dangerous and, in certain cases, fatal.

The Need for Micronutrients in a Vegetarian Diet

There is irony in calling vegetarianism a dietary fad because most of the human beings on our planet, for economic reasons, subsist chiefly on vegetable foods. Nevertheless, it was only recently that vegetarianism became popular with large numbers of Americans, as a means of improving health.

There are a number of advantages to vegetarianism. The Seventh-Day Adventists, who are vegetarians, have been found to have less cancer and heart disease than most other Americans. Fruits, vegetables, grains, beans, nuts and seeds contain all of the nutrients required to sustain animal life. They also contain fewer of the pollutants known to become concentrated in animal tissues at the top of the food chain since pesticides, hormones and antibiotics are all concentrated in animal tissues to a greater extent than in vegetables. Thus, a recent study found that the milk of nursing vegetarian mothers contained less pesticide residue than the milk of meat-eating nursing mothers.

In addition, vegetarianism is much less of a drain on the world food supply and may soon become an inevitable part of the American lifestyle as the price of meat goes out of sight. Perhaps the most persuasive feature of the vegetarian diet is that so many people "feel better," as they report it, on this diet than on any other. Now that we appreciate the value of crude fiber and trace minerals, which are abundantly supplied in vegetable matter, more and more of us are beginning to look critically at the concentrated, low-roughage meat and dairy foods.

On the other hand, there is no doubt that the protein value of vegetable foods is lower than animal foods. Not only is the quantity of protein low in vegetables, but so is its *quality*. Vegetable protein is less concentrated in the eight essential amino acids required by all animals for life. Only vegetables can manufacture these amino acids from inorganic chemicals, nitrogen, carbon dioxide and water, but it is animal flesh that concentrates them. If one follows a strict vegetarian diet, unless foods are properly combined *at the same meal* to complement these amino acids so that adequate amounts of all eight are present, the body is unable to use the rest. For example, wheat is low in the amino acid lysine while beans are low in methionine. The lowest level of any of the essential amino acids ingested is known as the limiting factor; only as much tissue can be built as is available from this "weakest link."

This is a very important point. I have seen many cases where vegetarians were ineffective at food combining. Often they feel well, even better than when on a complete diet of both animal and vegetable sources, but after a while the body is forced to steal amino acids from its own tissues, resulting in wasting of muscle and skin, often concealed by fat that remains intact while the body burns its proteins. When the ribs start to show, it is clearly time to correct protein deficiencies.

Therefore, the healthiest vegetarians are likely to be the ovo-lacto vegetarians, those who include eggs and milk products in their diet, while still shunning meat. Remember, eggs and milk provide the highest quality protein. Albumin and casein are the standards of completeness of amino acids. I recommend that some fish and occasional organ meat be included in the vegetarian lifestyle to assure complete nutrition. There are serious perils in even the most experienced vegetarian households, such as the Seventh-Day Adventists.

One of my patients was a thirty-seven-year-old vegetarian janitor, recently divorced. Deaf since infancy, his handicap kept him under stress. However, he had kept a job and been married for ten years. Then he suddenly became irritable, confused, and finally downright paranoid and delusional, thinking that his wife was carrying on behind his back and that someone was out to harm him. His wife left him, he lost his job, and his parents had to take him in to live under their care.

When I examined him and took his medical history I guessed at once that he might be deficient in vitamin B_{12} and the laboratory tests confirmed this. Vitamin B_{12} is the nutrient most likely to be lacking in a vegetarian diet. For those individuals who happen to have a higher-than-average requirement for this vitamin, the consequences can appear as degeneration of the spinal cord and brain cells. Usually, there is anemia also, as the blood cells do not form properly when there is a B_{12} deficiency. Although this patient did not have an actual anemia—that is, his liver still had enough stored B_{12} for the manufacture of blood cells—there was not enough for maintenance of the brain cells and transmitter substances. Within hours of his first injection of vitamin B_{12} he felt better, had more energy and was less depressed. Within two weeks he was fully rational and able to understand and dispel his delusions. Once the diagnosis was made, the cure was relatively simple. But for this man, the vegetarian diet had had tragic consequences just the same.

A more subtle complication of the vegetarian diet, especially one that does not include egg and milk products, is lack of methionine. This amino acid is necessary for the structure and function of every cell in your body. Many enzymes that control your body chemistry are made from it. Methionine deficiency becomes quickly evident in loss of energy, mood depression and loss of hair. Some of my patients have developed salt deficiencies. Lack of sodium and chloride in vegetables can be associated with fatigue and depression and in hot weather can be extremely dangerous. Salt depletion can develop in a few hours due to extra losses from sweating after heavy exercise and exposure to heat, as from being in a sauna. Don't forget that diuretic medications can also deplete salt. Beginning with muscle cramps and twitching, symptoms of salt depletion can worsen and eventually lead to damage to the heart and nervous system. Sunstroke and heat prostration are both related to salt depletion and are more likely to occur on a low-salt diet. Many vegetarians use soy sauce, which is high in salt, as a condiment.

I have measured the sodium and chloride levels in some of my vegetarian patients and found a few whose daily urine output was so low that they lacked sufficient chloride to form hydrochloric acid (hydrogen chloride) in the stomach. After increasing their salt intake they not only felt better but again secreted acid normally. As you can see, a vegetarian diet can be hazardous if not properly planned. I do not believe it is sensible to undertake such a dietary regimen unless you are prepared to study vegetarian nutrition thoroughly and follow the known principles of healthy vegetarianism consistently. In addition, it is not a bad idea to consult your physician for at least a yearly physical examination until you are sure that you have mastered your individual requirements.

The best-known reducing diets are analyzed in the following table. I have simply characterized the concept behind each diet and appended a comment or two on each method regarding the shortcomings. All of the reducing diets are low in calories. The proportions of protein, fat and carbohydrate as well as micronutrients, such as vitamins and minerals, differ from one diet method to another. Some are high in protein, others low; some are high in carbohydrate, others low; some are high in fat, most are low. Unfortunately, as you will notice, all of these reducing diets are also rather low in micronutrients. It is this feature that most urgently needs—and gets—attention in the orthocarbohydrate (OC) diet we will see in Chapter 15. This is, I feel, the most sensible and simplest way to lose weight without jeopardizing health. Since it is also based on the principles of determining proper carbohydrate levels, it also gives you a general guide to follow for feeling your absolute best, all of the time.

The Nutrition Prescription for Weight Loss or Gain

- Before going on a reducing diet, assure yourself of adequate micro-nutrients
- Become a nibbler instead of a gorger—small meals are best—but don't nibble any processed food
- Beware of any extreme in a diet, including some vegetarian diets, as they are lacking in nutrients
- Avoid sweeteners because they induce a craving for carbohydrates and foster self-indulgent habits of eating
- Don't rely on weight as a measure of nutrition, for it is possible to be overweight and undernourished
- Read Chapter 15, "The OC Diet," to individualize your diet program according to your needs

Diet Method	Protein	Fat	Carbohydrate	Micro-Nutrient
Total Fast	none	none	none	none

Comment: Weight loss slows because metabolic rate drops to low thyroid activity

Diet Method	Protein	Fat	Carbohydrate	Micro-Nutrient
Gonadotrophin Injections (HCG)	low	none	low	low

Comment: This diet is so low in calories and nutrients that it must be limited to only 3 weeks. The key to success for many people is the fact that it provides daily contact with the doctor or nurse, meals are precisely measured in prepared packages.

Diet Method	Protein	Fat	Carbohydrate	Micro-Nutrient
Juice Fast	low	none	moderate to high	low

Comment: Weight loss slows in a few days followed by weakness and hunger.

Diet Method	Protein	Fat	Carbohydrate	Micro-Nutrient
Scarsdale	moderate (40–50g)	low	low	low

Comment: Weight loss slows in a few weeks followed by weakness and hunger.

Diet Method	Protein	Fat	Carbohydrate	Micro-Nutrient
Liquid Protein	low	low	low	low

Comment: Incomplete and inadequate in nutrients. Dangerous.

Diet Method	Protein	Fat	Carbohydrate	Micro-Nutrient
Stillman Inches Off	low	low	moderate	low

Comment: Even Stillman says this diet should be limited to six weeks due to lack of nutrients. It is similar to a vegetarian fast.

Diet Method	Protein	Fat	Carbohydrate	Micro-Nutrient
Stillman Weight Loss	high	low	low	low

Comment: This diet causes ketosis, according to Stillman, and therefore must have more fat and less protein than indicated.

Diet Method	Protein	Fat	Carbohydrate	Micro-Nutrient
Atkins Low Carbohydrate	high	medium	low	medium

Comment: This diet is headed in the same general direction as the OC diet. (See Chapter 15)

4

Heart Disease: Causes, Correlations, Conspiracies

The first heart attack was classified and reported in 1896. For the next two decades the new disease got scant attention. After two world wars the Western world began to sense that it had a killer on its hands to rival the old enemies of mankind: pneumonia, influenza, smallpox. In the early fifties we learned that heart disease was not confined to the middle-aged and old: autopsies performed on soldiers in the Korean War showed advanced atherosclerosis in teenagers. By 1970 coronary heart disease had become the leading cause of death in America. Since 1973 the incidence of the disease has dropped 20 percent, though it still kills 600,000 Americans each year as a new decade begins. *Yet there is a good chance the last heart attack may be reported in our lifetime.*

The reason for my optimism is not that some other disease will take its place or that everyone will suddenly stop smoking, but that people who want to live past their prime will see that they have to change their way of *eating.* For the key to this twentieth-century phenomenon is clearly in our diet and how our diet is helped or hindered by our level of physical activity.

The disease I'm talking about has many names and symptoms. In the broadest terms, it is cardiovascular—affecting the heart and the blood vessels. Cardiovascular disease of all kinds accounts for more than half the deaths in the United States, about one million a year. In simplest terms, these deaths are all the result of a failure of blood to get to vital organs—to the brain (stroke) or to the heart (heart attack). Without the oxygen and many other nutrients that the blood carries, these organs die, wholly or partially. *Why* the blood fails to get to those organs distinguishes various diseases: a hardening of the arteries (atherosclerosis, or the equally descriptive name arteriosclerosis), a clotting of blood (thrombosis), or sudden stress on the heart muscle (angina pectoris). If the coronary arteries which encircle the heart like a crown are affected, the disease is called coronary heart disease. If blood fails to get to a portion of the heart and that muscle dies, it's called a myocardial infarction, the medical term for a heart attack. We can easily understand why the sudden stress of running up a flight of stairs can put a burden on the heart, but why do clots and other obstructions form in the arteries? The answer brings us to that most discussed of all villains, cholesterol—literally "hard bile," chemically in alcohol carried by lipoprotein, a fat/protein molecule, throughout the body. Cholesterol is sort of a "spare parts" source for the body's hormones. Its role in heart disease is critical and generally misunderstood. To see why, let's back up.

The "Diet of Commerce" Correlation

For the past two generations medical science has sought an explanation for this malady that seems to strike otherwise healthy young people in the prime of their lives. The first clue, and an obvious one, is the very fact that heart attacks are a twentieth-century disease. Does the cause lie in the conditions, the environment, of our age? The fast pace of civilization, the urbanization of our society, physical and emotional stress? No doubt these factors play a role: the serious-minded, competitive, Type A personality is known to be more susceptible to heart attacks. But is the stress of life in our time really that much greater than in previous centuries? I doubt it. If it were so, why does the incidence of coronary heart disease decline during wartime, especially under hardship conditions?

This is the second major clue: the rate of occurrence of heart attacks declines when wartime conditions dictate a return to a more primitive diet—whole grains and smaller amounts (due to shortages) of white flour, sugar and meat. When we study the effects of a primitive diet in almost every civilization on this planet, we find that there are no heart attacks. They occur only when the time-tested native diet, whatever its particular form, is replaced by a diet more suitable to mass production, ease of distribution, and shelf life than to the needs of the human body.

As long ago as the early 1920s, studies by the dentist-anthropologist Weston Price called attention to what has since been termed the "diet of commerce": staples that have all been refined to the point of actually looking alike—white flour, white rice, white sugar, white salt. His book, *Nutrition and Physical Degeneration,* was the first in a long series of denunciations of the spread of this diet throughout the modern world. Correlations have been made between the abandonment of native diets of almost any type and the near-epidemic increase in dental decay, diabetes, vascular disease, heart attacks, and cancer. Impressive as these correlations are, their very breadth has seemed to discourage any sort of corrective action other than much wringing of hands and an appeal to individuals to avoid the modern diet wherever possible.

In the case of heart disease, however, more specific correlations with diet have been attempted and have had an impact on public policy. Dr. Ancel Keys of the University of Minnesota pioneered in this work with studies of changes in dietary patterns in six countries during and after World War II. Higher intakes of fat and accompanying cholesterol before and after the war were correlated with surges in coronary heart disease (CHD). It was assumed that dietary cholesterol led inevitably to higher serum cholesterol in the blood and that serum cholesterol was therefore a cause of heart attacks.

It was also observed about this time that an increase in the intake of *vegetable* fats reduced serum cholesterol—perhaps because these fats replaced animal fats, perhaps because, as polyunsaturates, they had a positive effect on the reduction of cholesterol in the body. Physicians accordingly advised their patients against the saturated (hardened, saturated with hydrogen) fats or cholesterol present in meat, milk, butter and eggs. And they recommended various vegetable salad oils and soft margarines. The net result was a further push toward the diet of commerce, since the natural "farm" foods were eliminated from the diet. The message was simple enough, and it reached the man or woman in the street. Between 1940 and 1970 the per capita consumption of eggs and meat decreased one-third while the intake of polyunsaturates doubled. Yet as cholesterol in the diet was decreasing, heart attacks were on the rise.

The dietary cholesterol theory nevertheless gained support when a landmark study began in Massachusetts in 1950. More than 2000 people were observed over a 22-year period in the village of Framingham in a government-sponsored test of the serum cholesterol connection with heart disease. Early reports confirmed the correlation. By 1964, it seemed that the evidence was in: figures at 14 years into the study indicated a fourfold increase in heart attacks when the blood cholesterol was higher than 240 milligrams (per 100 milliliters of blood) and the risk went up to six times greater when the blood cholesterol was over 260 milligrams.

With odds like that, most Americans were easily persuaded to eat less meat, eggs, and cheese. The fact that previous studies had already demonstrated only a one-day rise in blood cholesterol after eating the equivalent of four dozen eggs at a single meal was curiously ignored. Not until 1975, when Dr. Roslyn Alfin-Slater and her colleagues at UCLA tested the effects of a normal diet with either one extra egg a day or two extra eggs a day (using healthy subjects and spreading the test over a two-month period), was it shown that there was no difference in the blood cholesterol level of subjects on these varying diets. It has been objected that these subjects were less sensitive to cholesterol in the diet to begin with, but the results are unexplainable by the cholesterol theory still in vogue.

The incontrovertible proof that eggs, which contain approximately 250 milligrams of cholesterol each, do not cause CHD was demonstrated in an analysis of diet and health conducted by Drs. Hammond and Garfinkel for the American Cancer Society. They studied 800,000 Americans for six years in the 1970s, grouping their observations into those eating fewer than five eggs a week compared to those eating five or more eggs a week. Their conclusion: those eating fewer eggs developed *more* heart disease.

Fats in the diet have been cleared as a direct cause of CHD for the great *majority* of people. (Some 10 percent of the population can handle neither fats nor salt nor even a minimum of sugar.) Throughout the world there are a number of societies where the native diet is high in fat and where CHD is rare or unknown. The Eskimos, the Masai, the Samburu, and the Yemenite Jews are a few examples.

Perhaps the most convincing study of this factor was done by Dr. S. L. Malhotra, who studied the incidence of CHD in railway sweepers in India. In northern India the diet is ten times higher in fat than in southern India. The northern diet is high in fresh and fermented milk (yogurt) while the southern diet is mostly vegetarian. Even though the northern Indians ate 10 times more fat and smoked 8 times more than their southern counterparts, the incidence of CHD was 15 times lower among northern Indians.

It seems a low-fat diet isn't sufficient in itself to prevent heart disease. Every one of the 10,000 autopsies performed at Dachau revealed the presence of atherosclerosis in blood vessels. A 1000-calorie-a-day diet (at most), low-fat intake, plenty of exercise, and hard labor were the conditions of the prisoners in the Dachau concentration camp. The serum cholesterol theory can't explain these epidemiological studies. My conclusion is that these atherosclerotic people—the concentration-camp Jews, the Indian railway sweepers, and the thousands of Americans in the Hammond–Garfinkel study—were deficient in certain anti-athero-sclerosis *micronutrients*.

The Cholesterol Mechanism

I well remember the impact that Dr. Keys' teachings had on me, for I was a medical student at the University of Minnesota in 1953 when his theory was introduced. Cholesterol had first been observed in athero-sclerotic plaque by the great pathologist Rudolph Virchow a century ear-lier and confirmed by Dr. Nikolai Anitschkow in 1913, so I assumed that the theory had already stood the test of time. Plaque is the fatty substance that restricts the blood vessels as it lodges in them. As choles-terol is "stockpiled" from overproduction it adheres to the intima (lin-ing) of the vessels, where it can cause clots to form. The question is: why is it overproduced?

I was particularly impressed with the Anitschkow experiments, which showed advanced atherosclerosis in rabbits fed high-cholesterol diets. Their blood cholesterol levels rose 10 to 20 times normal. What I didn't realize at that time was that the amounts of cholesterol used in the ex-periments were far in excess of what a rabbit would normally encounter in his diet, since rabbits are vegetarians. Also, a rabbit's atherosclerosis is different from that seen in human beings. The blood vessels and other tissues are filled to overflowing with fat in the rabbit, whereas in the human being atherosclerosis usually appears as cholesterol deposits (lo-calized plaques) that appear in response to apparent injury to the in-tima.

Further, I didn't learn until later that Dr. John Yudkin had shown an even higher correlation between CHD and dietary sugar than CHD and cholesterol. This makes good sense, for it is now known that eating sugar can induce diabetes (high blood sugar) in many people. High blood sugar levels produce sorbitol, an alcohol derivative of sugar, in our tissues. It is well established that sorbitol can migrate into blood vessel walls and damage cells, thus causing atherosclerosis, just as it can do in the lens of our eyes, causing cataracts. Both of these disorders are known to occur at a higher rate in diabetics. (Incidentally, there are good indications that this damage can be prevented by the administration of bioflavonoids, which prevent the conversion of blood glucose into sorbitol. Bioflavonoids are substances that accompany vitamin C and have never been considered important. In fact, the Nutrition Board has never wanted to accord them the status of "vitamins," even though they can save your eyes—or your life.)

The Micronutrient Effect and Lecithin

Does this mean that science has been wrong about cholesterol for over 30 years? Yes. The irony of the situation is that scientific advances have now put cholesterol in a new perspective and it is not all bad. In fact, as you may have guessed, cholesterol is just now beginning to be more appreciated. Many authorities ignore the fact that the cholesterol molecule is such a vital substance that almost every cell in the body manufactures it. This highly complex molecule is the raw material out of which your body makes vitamin D, which helps regulate your calcium levels. It is also the source for the important steroid hormones of the body: the sex hormones and the stress hormones both come from cholesterol. Cholesterol is also necessary for the manufacture of bile in the liver. Thus it is absolutely needed to promote emulsification and absorption of fat and so is indirectly required for adequate absorption of fat-soluble nutrients, such as vitamins A, D, E, and K.

Your cholesterol level will remain essentially unaffected by a low-cholesterol diet because the body manufactures the substance if it is not ingested. Blood cholesterol is actively regulated by a feedback mechanism so that when the dietary intake of cholesterol increases, the liver manufactures less of it. The amount actually manufactured in the body is from 1,000 to 2,000 milligrams per day. This compares to an average of about 500 milligrams in your diet. (Each egg accounts for about 250 milligrams, a ¼-pound portion of liver about the same, and an equal amount of shellfish about half as much.) Other meats have weight for weight about a third the cholesterol found in liver. An ounce of butter has as much as an ounce of liver, about 70 milligrams.

For those who can handle cholesterol—perhaps 90 percent of the population—a large dietary intake has another positive aspect. The manufacture of cholesterol in the body requires energy and micronutrients. It is made from acetate, co-enzyme A, and pantothenic acid, among other elements. It is conceivable that by ingesting a substantial amount of dietary cholesterol, the liver actually is relieved of some chemical work and can use its chemical energies for other functions, such as regulating the nutrient supply of the blood and detoxifying environmental pollutants.

A deficiency of cholesterol is not necessarily a sign of good health. In fact, *low* cholesterol can be a sign of starvation, comparable to such signals as weakness and vulnerability to disease. Deficiencies of vitamin A and of the mineral manganese are commonly associated with very low levels of cholesterol (under 130 milligrams). On the other hand, very high levels of cholesterol, over 300 milligrams, may indicate interference with the body's ability to excrete the molecule. Stress induces increased cholesterol synthesis. This may account for the higher incidence of CHD in Dr. Friedman's Type A men. In addition, stress depletes the body of vitamin C; this can be even more important. As Dr. Carlos Krumdieck and Charles Butterworth point out in their analysis of the problem: "Vitamin C seems to occupy a position of unique importance by virtue of its involvement in two systems: the maintenance of vascular integrity and the metabolism of cholesterol in bile acids." When vitamin C is deficient, cholesterol cannot be removed normally from the blood as it passes through the liver. This causes a bottleneck in cholesterol excretion and forces cholesterol levels to go up in the blood. That which does get excreted in the bile may be incompletely soluble and is liable to form gallstones. Cholesterol is named from the Greek words meaning "hard bile."

While vitamin C is required by the liver to remove cholesterol from the blood, lecithin is necessary to make cholesterol soluble and remove it from the tissues and artery walls so that it can be transported by the high-density lipoproteins (HDL) to the liver. Only lecithins made from unsaturated fats can perform this job; hence the advantage of vegetable oils over animal fats. Even the lecithin from eggs is incapable of removing cholesterol, for it has the wrong type of unsaturated fat, unable to attach to the cholesterol and make it soluble. Deficiency in dietary unsaturated fats or lecithin permits cholesterol to pile up in the tissues and remain there—unless the body has sufficient vitamin B_6, magnesium, and other micronutrients from which to make its own lecithin to do the job.

Thus, cholesterol deposits in the blood vessel walls do predispose to the formation of plaque, narrowing of the blood vessel channels and accumulation of clots on the damaged areas. This can block circulation and provoke heart attacks and strokes. However, cholesterol is clearly not alone as a risk to your blood vessels. Toxic materials that form free radicals, such as cigarette smoke and chlorinated water, can also cause damage to cells in the blood vessels. In addition, they deplete micronutrients, such as vitamins C and E, which are used up in neutralizing the free radicals. *Deficiency of these and other micronutrients are, in my opinion, the most important causes of atherosclerosis and CHD.*

Both vitamin E and vitamin C are protective against free radical damage to the cells in the blood vessels, which is now believed to be the most important cause of atherosclerosis. The mineral selenium activates an enzyme that gives further protection. The mineral copper is also essential, for it is involved with vitamin C in the manufacture of collagen, the protein of which blood vessels are made. Vitamin E is also known to protect against unwanted blood clotting. If the body stores of vitamin E are low, vitamin C is used to regenerate and conserve E. As you can see, these two vital nutrients work as a team, but other vitamins and minerals are also important. Deficiency of both zinc and copper have been detected in atherosclerotic vessels, and magnesium deficiency in the heart muscle is often associated with fatal heart attacks. Deficiency of vitamin B_6 is important, not only for the production of lecithin but also to protect against the toxic effects of the amino acid homocysteine, a known cause of atherosclerosis, and highly suspect in those who consume excess protein in their diet. Finally, chromium is essential to regulate blood sugar and prevent diabetes. High blood sugar levels actually damage the blood vessel cells and cause atherosclerosis.

Low-Cholesterol Conspiracies

Dr. Roger J. Williams, the discoverer of the important B vitamin, pantothenic acid, says, "I am convinced the avoidance of cholesterol-containing foods is most unfortunate because the very best foods we have contain more cholesterol than do the less nutritious foods. I also have the strong impression . . . that if we get into our systems a good assortment of essential nutrients, the matter of cholesterol, saturated fats and unsaturated fats will pretty much take care of itself."

Dr. George V. Mann, of the Vanderbilt University School of Medicine, published a landmark article, "Cholesterol: End of an Era," in September 1977 in the *New England Journal of Medicine*. He commented, "Galileo would have flinched if he had observed the pseudo-scientific procedures of the American Heart Association regarding the cholesterol 'propaganda.'" The scientific issues, he said, were being settled by "majority vote," adding that dietary research was "busywork for thousands of chemists," and that to be a dissenter was "to be unfunded because the peer review system rewards conformity and excludes criticism." His review of the data demolishing the dietary cholesterol theory of CHD remains essentially unchallenged.

At the same time, a United States Senate committee on nutrition laid down this recommendation to the nation: "Reduce cholesterol consumption to about 300 milligrams per day." Nor have other semiofficial bodies gotten the message. The Center for Science in the Public Interest (CSPI), a privately funded organization in Washington, D.C., continues to push for a low-cholesterol diet with warnings against consumption of eggs, butter, and whole milk. The American Heart Association has relaxed its strictures against dietary fat only to the extent of emphasizing exercise more than it has ever done. When responsible organizations like these find it difficult to recognize the fact that the old cholesterol theory was wrong, how can we expect the layperson to adjust to the new evidence—even when the evidence is presented in convincing fashion? Our cholesterol phobia is so great that it will be years before the public will again fully accept such foods as butter, eggs, and milk.

There is obviously much at stake for manufacturers of vegetable oils, as well as for the egg industry. When the evidence seems to run against them, both sides in this nutritional tug-of-war cite the economic motive of the opposition. And so we have allegations of conspiracies, for the research efforts on both sides are often funded by groups which stand to benefit from favorable verdicts for their products. It's time to put aside these political attacks and listen to the evidence: for the broad public, cholesterol in food is not the problem.

Beware the Easy Answer, Beware the Extremes

It simply doesn't make sense that a staple of human consumption for eons, animal fat, should turn out to be the cause of a sudden increase in human maladies in less than a century. There is a complexity of biochemical and nutritional factors involved in maintaining health and in preventing such disasters as heart attacks. Multiple factors are the rule in any medical question, not least in nutrition; and multiple nutrients are critical in heart disease.

Now we can come back to the epidemic proportions of cardiovascular disease cited at the beginning of this chapter. Three major changes in the environment—about 30 years apart from each other—suggest why this century ushered in heart attacks. These changes were essentially dietary: (1) the introduction of refined and bleached flour; (2) large-scale chlorination of water supplies; and (3) homogenization of milk. All three contributed; no single factor is the villain. This is why you will read from time to time that enriched white bread isn't all that bad, even though it's not as good as whole-wheat bread. True. But you don't have to become a faddist of any kind to recognize that the accumulation of dietary deficiencies from a variety of sources can be just as bad as a single, gross dietary mistake.

In the technological advance of milling flour, the wheat germ is systematically stripped from the grain, along with the B vitamins, vitamin E, and such trace metals as magnesium, manganese, and chromium. It took nearly a century for the country's health authorities to wake up to the fact that nutrient-deficiency diseases such as pellagra, beriberi, anemia, and a variety of unnamed syndromes resulting from lack of multiple B vitamins might be due to milling flour. In 1941 a federal agency mandated the enrichment of white flour with B_1, B_2, B_3, and the mineral iron. No one made a connection at the time between these and other vitamins and minerals on the one hand and heart disease on the other. As we have seen, even today the cholesterol chant drowns out the message about micronutrients. The so-called enrichment of bread, however, was really just spare change.

Three of the B vitamins and one readily available mineral were put back after twenty vitamins and minerals were removed. The authorities weren't penurious; they simply didn't know at the time about the vital roles of the vitamins E, B_6, and folic acid and the whole range of trace minerals. (You may have noticed that as recently as the late 1970s labels on vitamin E bottles stated that there was no established nutritional role for it.)

All right. That was almost 40 years ago. Knowing what we do now, what are the millers enriching our flour with? Read the label on your bread wrapper: thiamine (vitamin B_1), riboflavin (vitamin B_2), niacin (vitamin B_3), and iron. That's it. Oh yes: the shortening is probably hydrogenated vegetable oil, a "trans" or transformed fat that has recently been pinpointed as a suspect in cardiovascular disease. The flour industry is something like the tax collectors of modern government—

once they've taken something away, never expect anything but a trickle back.

Thirty years after we had become accustomed to white bread on the table, along came a second precursor of heart disease. In 1910, our water supplies began to be treated with chlorine, a chemical that kills germs even in water standing in pipes. This public health measure was widely adopted throughout the country; today there are 40,000 or more municipal water districts in the United States and all their supplies are chlorinated. Again, it wasn't known then, and is scarcely mentioned now, that even in the minute quantities sufficient to kill germs, chlorine can undermine the body's defenses against atherosclerosis. Chlorine creates electrically charged molecules called free radicals, which can combine with alpha tocopherol (vitamin E) and eliminate it from your system. In addition, free radicals can directly damage the intima of blood vessels and so create the environment for the formation of plaques. It's now being recognized that chlorine is dangerous enough to be considered a pollutant; and perhaps this fact in itself will prove to be a blessing. Chlorine has been found to interact with industrial wastes in water to produce carcinogens; as we will see in the next chapter, the threat of cancer is perhaps the only mega-micronutritional factor strong enough in the public consciousness to effect a change in public policy.

Incidentally, the depletion of vitamin E in milled flour and in chlorinated water is bad enough without another ominous trend. Linus Pauling points out that the price of vitamin E has gotten so high—nearly $100 per kilogram as compared with $7.50 per kilogram for vitamin C—that food companies are now stripping E from vegetable oils to sell it separately. This lowers vitamin E in your diet.

You can avoid white bread, but what about chlorinated water? Pauling suggests that a pinch of vitamin C crystals in a glass of water removes residual chlorine by chemical combination. Easier yet is to let your drinking water stand in an open container at room temperature for half a day; the chlorine will evaporate. Or boil your water, as if you were in a strange locale where the purity of the water is uncertain. You can also invest in a home distillation system. In our so-called modern society, all of this may seem ludicrous; and, as in the case of the "diet of commerce," chlorine alone is not the villain. But until a logical successor to chlorine is found (ozone treatment works at the water plant but not in the pipes), our drinking water will continue to be a contributing factor to heart disease.

Finally, some 30 years after widespread chlorination of our water supply began, a third dietary change occurred in this country that would further weaken our protection against atherosclerosis, the homogenization of milk. The homogenized fat droplets bypass the liver and are absorbed directly into the lymphatic system and then into the bloodstream.

There is an enzyme in cow's milk, xanthine oxidase, which is known to irritate the lining of blood vessels. If this xanthine oxidase enzyme were not carried by the homogenized fat droplets in milk, it would be eliminated by chemical action in the body's protector, the liver.

Thus we are faced with the dilemma of drinking homogenized whole milk, with its wide variety of nutrients, and thereby also ingesting xanthine oxidase in a dangerous form. This is the best argument for drinking low-fat milk. Or you can heat your milk to 92°C for 5 seconds to inactivate the enzyme. Dr. Kurt Oster has concluded that the 70 percent rate of atherosclerosis in American soldiers in the Korean War (average age at autopsy: twenty-two) is accounted for only by a drastic change in diet from World War I to II. Despite the prevalence of white bread and chlorinated water during those wars, autopsies showed little atherosclerosis in soldiers up to 1945. The villain: xanthine oxidase carried by homogenized fat droplets.

Cholesterol Doesn't Count?

In any discussion of complex dietary health issues, we must remind ourselves not to run to extreme positions. This is one of the implications in the term "orthomolecular," which means the right amounts of the right molecules—in a word: optimum. The bottom line on cholesterol, then, is this: What is the optimal range of serum cholesterol that is right for you? At most laboratories in the United States anywhere from 160 to 300 milligrams per 100 milliliters of blood is considered normal. However, the Framingham study showed a fourfold increase of CHD in men with serum cholesterol over 240. On the other hand, Dr. William Castelli and Mr. Nathan Pritikin claim there is virtually no CHD with serum cholesterol under 150. This sounds very persuasive until we find that in Japan, Dr. Hirotsuga Ueshima reports from the Department of Epidemiology for Cardiovascular Diseases that as the serum cholesterol drops below 200 the rate of occurrence of stroke increases and below 160 the rate of mortality from cerebral hemorrhage also increases. While a very low fat and cholesterol intake will usually result in these low levels of serum cholesterol, they may also cause inadequate absorption of fat-soluble vitamins, such as vitamins A, D, E, and K. In certain impoverished countries people survive on a necessarily low-fat diet. It is not optimal, for there is a serious problem of vitamin A deficiency, causing permanent blindness in tens of thousands of children in Africa.

Before you throw caution to the winds, however, and disregard serum cholesterol, be advised that high cholesterol is, indeed, a risk factor for CHD and cancer. Serum cholesterol above 260 is statistically a hazard. That means the odds of danger increase even though many individuals can tolerate such high levels without bad effects. Remember also that the statistics which indict high serum cholesterol as a cause of CHD are based on research in which no attention was paid to nutritional status. Now that we know that vitamin C and other nutrients offer protection against this hazard, the Framingham study is obsolete. I think it is very likely that the 20 percent drop in CHD in this country since 1970 is in fact due to the increasing use of megadose ascorbate. As the sales of vitamin C have gone up, the rate of CHD has gone down.

The Nutrition Prescription for the Heart Disease–Cholesterol Controversy

- Stop worrying about dietary cholesterol if your micronutrients are adequate; no need to avoid eggs, liver, cheese, and butter
- If you do favor a high fat intake, extra amounts of vitamins E and C are required
- Of all the factors that have been associated with CHD, excess body fat is most reliably established. Of all the treatments that have been able to lower serum cholesterol and improve atherosclerosis, again weight reduction stands out—but it must be accompanied with replenishment of the vital micronutrients
- If you do have a high serum cholesterol, it may be that you are overloaded with calories, undersupplied with nutrients, and getting too little exercise.

5

Let Your Heart Be Your Guide

Few things have wreaked as much havoc on the American diet (in addition to sheer negligence) as the search for extreme answers to the danger of heart disease. Millions of Americans now avoid some of the most nutritious, whole foods out of fear of dietary cholesterol. Others are willing to undertake a rigorous, ultra-low-fat regimen because of its success in rehabilitating apparently hopeless cardiac patients. My position is that any drastic change in diet that has not worked well over long periods of time is (1) contrary to common sense and (2) so stressful that it shouldn't be prolonged with the best of will power. Let's be sensible about our heart: as the central part of our body it must respond favorably to sound nutrition. Conversely, whatever we do that's good for the heart must be a pretty good guide to the rest of our health.

Here are some key rules and specific recommendations for the health of your heart; you will find them excellent guides for any lifestyle.

- Be sure to obtain adequate amounts of vitamins C, E, B_6 and minerals magnesium, selenium, and chromium.
- Avoid sugar and refined carbohydrates (especially the whites: white rice, white bread and white sugar) because they deplete the body of nutrients.
- Avoid salted foods because excessive salt can trigger arrhythmias.

- Avoid excess fats because of the ease with which they overload the body chemistry.
- Eat more frequently and take smaller portions: Six small meals a day instead of three will keep the blood sugar more stable.
- Eat more vegetables, such as nuts, seeds, whole grains, potatoes, sweet potatoes, carrots, salad vegetables, berries, and only two fruits a day for micronutrients and fiber.
- Eat more low-fat animal foods, such as fish, fowl (skinned), shellfish, liver, kidney and sweetbreads; eat yogurt, cottage cheese, and ricotta cheese.
- Eat up to two eggs a day as part of your diet despite their fat content.

These eight rules constitute something of a philosophy of eating and exercise that I call mega-nutrition. Because it is a philosophy and not a magic formula or crash diet, it must be tried and evaluated, not just copied down and played with. This chapter, then, is a summation of this book from another point of view: if you are concerned about your heart because of hereditary factors or personal history, this is an excellent way to become conversant with mega-nutrition.

Heart Rule No. 1: Get Your Micronutrients

This is a good place to bring up the subject of our knowledge of vitamins. We actually know more about the function of vitamins and minerals in the body than about virtually any other physiologically observable event. We know that vitamins work like a light dimmer, not only on or off, but in degrees of brightness. A minute difference in dosage can result in wide variations in mood or well-being. The vitamin taker is often rightly pictured as someone who gulps them down indiscriminately: a natural tendency is to assume that if a little of something is good, a lot will be even better. In the case of heart disease prevention, however, our first concern is to meet minimum requirements.

A deficiency of almost *any* micronutrient, in fact, can produce atherosclerosis. The vitamins C, E, A, and B_6 and the minerals chromium, selenium, zinc, and magnesium are most important. Nor are these nutrients simply insurance against dietary abuses in the system. That is, it's not true that these micronutrients simply protect you against a cholesterol-rich diet; they're needed whether you have a lot of dietary fat or not. Dr. Carl Pfeiffer says, "Although it is widely known that animals fed a diet high in cholesterol and saturated fats will develop atherosclerosis, the same is not true for human beings if adequate amounts of other nutrients, such as zinc and chromium and vitamin C, are also ingested." I would add that we need plenty of nutrients even if we don't have a diet high in fat.

The importance of micronutrition was amply demonstrated in the case of Patrick, a highly regarded career military officer until a heart attack at age fifty-two forced him to retire. He had suffered from an irregular pulse for years, which persisted despite medication. Bypass surgery was not recommended after his attack, in view of the fact that his angiogram showed that his coronary arteries were badly damaged by atherosclerosis. His wife, who was also in poor health, had been consulting me; she did so well on a micronutrition program that she persuaded her husband to take some of her nutrient supplements.

Although he was skeptical of supplements, Patrick went along with her. To his growing amazement, not only did he feel much better after a short time, but his pulse became more regular. After a year of continued improvement he was able to discontinue some of his heart pills and reduce the others. But there was still some arrhythmia.

At this point, he came to me for a checkup. He was not overweight. His cholesterol and HDL levels were normal. This implied only an average risk of CHD. His hair analysis, however, was quite revealing: very low levels of magnesium, zinc, calcium, and phosphorus. After dietary adjustments in these minerals, his heartbeat became steady for the first time in years and he was able to go back to work as an executive.

An old friend of mine learned about mega-nutrition under the same kind of circumstances. A talented artist, he is also very definitely a Type A personality: competitive, aggressive, impatient. This combination of traits in itself often leads to self-induced stress and an above-average risk of CHD. To make things worse, he was a two-pack-a-day smoker, he was careless about his food habits, and he was overweight. Suddenly, at age forty-six, he began to experience episodes of chest pain. Before long he was unable to walk more than a hundred feet before shortness of breath and choking, crushing chest pain stopped him.

His cardiology team wasted no time in working him up for bypass surgery. However, the X-ray angiograms showed all three coronary arteries seriously blocked by atherosclerotic plaques. He was advised that it was too late and too risky for surgery. His life expectancy was measured in months.

Desperate and depressed, he consulted me immediately after he got his X-ray report. After reviewing the data, I advised him to try an aggressive mega-nutrition program of the major vitamins and trace minerals, especially E and C. There was nothing to lose and maybe everything to gain.

Within only two weeks he was better and able to increase his walking exercise to two blocks. In a month he was getting around normally. He had stopped smoking, of course, and had cut out empty calories, such as white bread and sugar, replacing them with whole-wheat bread, vegetable salads, and spring water. He has never been one to jog or exercise vigorously since the onset of his chest pain, but he certainly walked enough. Now when he visits me in my study—seven years later—he climbs three flights of stairs at the same pace as I do, two stairs at a time.

The Untold Story of Trace Minerals

While the role of vitamins has been widely appreciated for many years, the importance of minerals that act as cofactors in directing chemical reactions in the body has only recently begun to receive attention. There is much yet to be learned, but it's quite certain that all the vitamins seem to require minerals in order to be effective in the chemistry of the cells. Thus, zinc combines with vitamin A to promote protein synthesis in cells, without which healing does not proceed properly. So it's highly interesting that zinc deficiency has been found in the aortas of patients who have died from CHD. In similar fashion, selenium is known to interact with vitamin E to protect the cell membranes from free radicals, thus preventing one of the common types of blood vessel damage that causes atherosclerosis. Vitamin C is ineffective as an antioxidant and builder of connective tissue unless copper is also present to act as a catalyst for the removal of two hydrogen molecules from the ascorbic acid molecule, which then combine with oxygen to become an extra molecule of water in the tissues.

According to Richard Passwater, in *Supernutrition for Healthy Hearts,* vitamin E and selenium are the most significant deficiencies in heart disease, more critical than vitamin C. I feel that all are equally vital. As long ago as 1953, Dr. G. C. Willis concluded that a deficiency of vitamin C in the arterial wall could lead to damage to the intima, or lining, and to the deposit of plaques. He tested this theory by measuring the amount of ascorbate in human aortas at autopsy: he found localized depletion of vitamin C in regions subjected to mechanical stress. This makes sense because these areas would be more active, rebuilding the collagen fibers and hence using up more vitamin C. Willis went on to study experimental atherosclerosis in guinea pigs, which, like ourselves, are unable to manufacture ascorbate. He found that subclinical vitamin C deficiency, not enough to cause scurvy, would cause atherosclerosis. It's a reasonable assumption that the same mechanism applies in the case of human beings.

It's worth reviewing the case for ascorbate in heart disease to show the interrelation of vitamins and minerals. Dr. Willis went on to demonstrate that vitamin C supplementation would reverse the damage from a prior period of vitamin C deprivation in guinea pigs. Then he studied ten patients, who had generalized atherosclerosis, by X-ray arteriograms of their legs. Partial removal of plaque occurred in six of ten patients who received 15 grams of vitamin C per day. None of the untreated comparison group improved. This conclusive work was done in the 1950's and somehow got brushed aside by the priority of the day: cholesterol. The irony is that it is now well established that vitamin C is also active in controlling blood cholesterol.

In 1971, Dr. Takao Fujinami fed guinea pigs coconut oil and varying amounts of vitamin C. After two weeks, elevation of blood cholesterol was found in the low-ascorbate group but not in the high-ascorbate group. The high cholesterol levels returned to normal in the low-ascorbate group when vitamin C was then increased. Dr. Fujinami concluded that the requirement for vitamin C may increase in relation to the amount of fat in the diet.

The researches of Emil Ginter, of the Institute of Human Nutrition in Bratislava, Czechoslovakia, indicate that the conversion of cholesterol to bile acids in the liver requires vitamin C. Without significant vitamin C, cholesterol remains insoluble. It will not be excreted efficiently and it is much more liable to form gallstones. Hard bile can mean gallstones as well as atherosclerosis unless vitamin C is amply supplied.

While copper has not yet been carefully studied in relation to atherosclerosis, it is well known that copper deficiency in animals leads to fibrosis of the heart and rupture of the aorta due to loss of elasticity. In 1974, Drs. B. and J. R. Chipperfield found copper deficiencies in the heart muscle of patients dying from heart attacks—at some time after the original attack.

In the same study, magnesium was also found deficient. This is important because magnesium is essential for the cell membrane in response to insulin, to activate most of the glucose energy reactions in the cells. Magnesium is also known to keep potassium in balance, thus pre-

serving the electrical energy of the cell. Finally, magnesium is in delicate balance with calcium, which also affects muscle contractility. Too
much calcium and too little magnesium may mean muscle cramp—or
heart stoppage.

As long ago as 1961, Dr. Frederick Stare, one of the more conservative nutrition authorities, reported that increasing dietary magnesium
in experiments with rats lowered the level of cholesterol. Even before
that, in 1957, Dr. J. J. Vitale discovered that when rats were fed a diet
with extra saturated fat, in the form of hydrogenated cottonseed oil and
cholesterol, the need for magnesium was increased up to 16 times. That
is, by increasing the dietary magnesium the expected fat deposits in the
heart were prevented. Other researchers confirmed this finding and
concluded that a magnesium deficiency would produce plaque in six
months to a year in human subjects.

One of the more exciting papers in 1974 was a report on heart disease by Dr. James Pershing Isaacs of Johns Hopkins School of Medicine, a pioneer in theory and practice of orthomedicine. He had treated
25 patients, all of whom had had at least one heart attack, with supplements of vitamin E, vitamin C, zinc, copper, and manganese. In addition, he had included a small dose of thyroid, which is known to lower
cholesterol. After ten years the benefits were gratifying in the extreme:
only 2 patients had died rather than the 13 who would have been expected to by the actuaries.

The foregoing discussion has focused on protection of the heart
blood vessels in particular, but let's not overlook the importance of the
blood itself in CHD. It's well known that some people with advanced
atherosclerosis remain healthy and well, while others get heart attacks,
leg pains, and phlebitis. Vitamin E may make the difference. In 1949,
Dr. Alton Ochsner, founder of the Ochsner Clinic and one of this country's most famous surgeons, found that vitamin E worked well in preventing blood clots. He reported, "The great advantage of using vitamin
E is that although the thrombosis tendency is overcome, a hemorrhagic
tendency is not produced such as occurs when anticoagulants . . . are
used." In 1972, Dr. K. Korsan Bengsten and his group of research colleagues observed a longer clotting time in patients recovering from heart
attacks when they were given 300 units of vitamin E daily. Other inves-
tigations have verified that vitamin E reduces the stickiness of blood
platelets, the tiny cells that initiate about 50 percent of all blood clots.
Selenium not only enhances the activity of vitamin E but also inde-

pendently activates an enzyme that protects cell membranes against injury by free radicals.

Of all the micronutrients tested in CHD, niacin (vitamin B_3) is best known. Dr. Abram Hoffer, one of the pioneers in megavitamin therapy for schizophrenia, discovered 20 years ago that a significant reduction in cholesterol is accomplished by this one vitamin alone. A five-year study of megadose niacin treatment in CHD showed a slight reduction in the number of repeat heart attacks. The fact that niacin, at doses as low as 50 to 100 milligrams, reduces platelet clumps and promotes capillary circulation gives it a definite place in micronutrient therapy of CHD.

Platelet clumping causes thrombosis by providing a footing in which fibrin can adhere and clog an artery. Vitamin E, at doses up to 1,800 units per day, has been observed to reduce platelet clumping by half. This is why vitamin E is considered by Dr. Passwater to be the most important step in preventing heart attacks.

Passwater's research is unusual and extensive. In a survey of almost 18,000 people between the ages of fifty and ninety-eight, of whom 20 percent had heart disease, he found that more than 80 percent reported that vitamin E helped their heart disease measurably. That is, fewer nitroglycerin pills were needed to control angina pains and, if the vitamins were stopped, the pains recurred. In addition, Dr. Passwater's study shows that vitamin E has a direct role in prevention of heart disease: in any age group the amount of heart disease decreased as the length of time that the vitamin had been taken increased.

For example, of 2,500 people who had taken vitamin E at a daily dose of 400 units or more for more than ten years, only four cases of CHD were found. Remember, these were people between ages fifty and ninety-eight. Statistical experience says that about *one-third* of that sample would experience some occurrence of heart disease at this age level. One-third of 2,500 people would be more than 800 cases of heart disease. The four cases therefore represented a reduction of CHD by two hundredfold!

Heart Rule No. 2: Exercise

The current popularity of active sports, particularly tennis and jogging, has given scientists a new population of human specimens to study in their search for causal relationships in CHD. Marathon runners, for example, have exhibited considerable immunity to atherosclerosis.

Could this be because long-distance runners work off more calories and hence eat more food and get more micronutrients? Or might it be that runners tend to be unusually aware of their nutritional needs, take more care of their diets and take extra vitamins C and E? Many authorities, including Dr. W. P. Castelli, director of laboratory research in the Framingham study, have observed the high levels of HDL cholesterol among marathon runners and joggers. As we have seen in Chapter 4, HDL is a critical protecting factor in CHD.

Dr. E. H. Hartung, assistant professor of physical medicine at Baylor College, found that even moderate jogging lowers cholesterol and tryglyceride levels and increases HDL, high-density lipoproteins, perhaps by helping remove the low-density lipoproteins from the body. In a study of 59 marathon runners, a 20 percent reduction in cholesterol was found in comparison to a group of inactive men with similar diets and habits. Even low-mileage runners studied at the same time did not get the same cholesterol-lowering effect but did get an increase in HDL.

A word of caution about overexercising is certainly appropriate for anyone planning to improve health habits. Remember, it takes weeks and months of conditioning to prepare your blood vessels and your body chemistry for the increased work load involved in these sports. To build up your exercise tolerance safely, I recommend that you read such books as *The New Aerobics* by Dr. Kenneth Cooper. I personally know of a number of people who have had fatal heart stoppage while jogging. In fact, this was recently the subject of a letter to the *Journal of the AMA* by a doctor who urged his colleagues to keep identification in their pockets if they intended to jog so that they could be identified if brought into an emergency room!

Another point worth emphasizing regarding exercise and mega-nutrition is the simple fact that exercise means energy is being used up. By using up energy *we increase the adaptive enzymes of the body chemistry,* which is good. However, if we use up more energy and micronutrients, we must also provide more in food. Extra amounts of potassium and magnesium are particularly important because it is well known that these are readily depleted in habitual exercisers. However, don't neglect salt if you sweat a lot. Leg cramps are good indicators that you need more potassium or sodium or both. A potassium-sodium mixture such as Morton's "Lite" salt, or other salt substitutes, taken in your tomato juice before jogging isn't a bad idea, because it assures you are getting both minerals in good proportion.

An additional important factor in active exercise is that it definitely increases the need for carbohydrate and lowers the need for fat. In fact, a high fat intake is usually considered uncomfortable by runners. Complex carbohydrates, in the form of whole-grain cereals and various beans and legumes, in addition to starch from potatoes and sweet potatoes, are preferred for priming the liver with the stored carbohydrate, glycogen. (Glycogen is the substance that is stored from the consumption of the basic energy source, carbohydrates. Elsewhere I have pointed out that active people feel best at higher levels of carbohydrate intake; see Chapter 15.) Smaller carbohydrates, in the form of fruits, berries, and melons, are good for a quick pickup after or during activity.

There are also medical authorities on diet who recommend that runners should avoid fat. Dr. Julian Whitaker, medical director of the Heart Center in San Clemente, California, has emphasized that when fat makes up more than 15 percent of dietary calories, the fat enters the bloodstream and fat droplets coat the red blood cells, which stick together like stacks of poker chips. These big clumps of red cells do not flow as well through the capillaries, reducing oxygen supply by up to 30 percent. Research in this field was originally done by Dr. Meyer Friedman. Recently, Dr. Per Olof Astrand observed that endurance on a stress test is three times greater on a high-carbohydrate, low-fat diet compared to a high-protein, high-fat diet.

The interrelationship of food and exercise is stronger than one would expect, even from reading any of the currently popular books and magazines on running and jogging. Experienced marathon runners have suffered serious illnesses after long training periods, not realizing the cumulative depletion of critical minerals this sport entails. Nutrition should not be used simply as a device to "get up" for that big race, the way carbohydrate "loading" is used by long-distance runners.

There are essentially two kinds of exercise: recreational and endurance. The former tolerates quite a bit of fat in the diet. But fat works against the endurance athlete, in two ways: fat emulsions coat blood cells and thus reduce oxygen delivery, and fat interferes with the release of glycogen from storage. This is the major reason why aerobic exercise leads to significant weight loss: it disposes one not to want fat in the diet.

Endurance or aerobic exercise calls for several mineral replacements, especially potassium. Several commercial drinks have been developed just for this purpose. Tomato juice, salted to taste, is therefore an excellent after-exercise drink, and orange juice (for its fructose/glucose as well as potassium) is a good before-exercise drink.

What is the place of protein in exercise? Aerobic workouts deplete the amino acids, and so they too have to be replaced since they can't be stored to any degree. Thus products that provide a predigested amino acid source have been developed for athletes who find it uncomfortable or impossible to eat before vigorous exercise. For the same reason, Dr. Tom Bassler recommends the intake of an egg for every six miles of running or walking. Finally, the antioxidants, vitamins C, E, and B_{15}, are important to reduce stress and maintain tissue strength. Consider especially the role of fiber and trace minerals (Chapter 11), such as are found in alfalfa, in building strong joints and collagen.

Heart Rule No. 3: Don't Smoke

When I was a young boy it was still considered rather tongue-in-cheek to tell a youngster that smoking would stunt his growth. Forty years later, it is no longer a joking matter. Now we know for certain that when the Surgeon General says cigarette smoking "may be hazardous to your health," he is understating the case. Smoking is perhaps the major hazard to your health. It is an environmental pollutant, not only for those who smoke, but for those who have to inhale the smoke-polluted air secondhand. Carbon monoxide and tars are certainly the most dangerous by-products of smoking, but for the smoker who inhales, significant amounts of cadmium (which can raise the blood pressure) and lead and arsenic (which can interfere with vital enzymes) must take their toll. The statisticians tell us that each "coffin nail" takes three minutes off a life.

The risk of heart attack is significantly increased in smokers and is proportional to the number of cigarettes smoked. The National Cooperative Pooling Project cited a study of CHD in 11,000 men which found that the risk of a first heart attack was 18 per 1,000 for men in their fifties who smoked more than a pack a day. Nonsmokers and those who had quit smoking had a risk of 3 per 1,000, or six times less.

Recently, Drs. Bain, Hennekens, and Rosner of the Harvard Medical School found that merely reducing cigarette smoking from over two packs a day to between one and two packs a day will reduce the risk of CHD by half. If smoking is cut in half again, to less than a pack a day, the risk is cut in half once more. In other words, heavy smokers have four times the risk of heart attack than light smokers.

Do you still want a cigarette?

Heart Rule No. 4: Maintain Your Optimal Weight

Despite thousands of scientific studies throughout the world, there is no conclusive proof that dietary fat is of itself a cause of CHD. On the other hand, there is very definite proof that *excess body fat,* obesity, is correlated with CHD. Since approximately half of all adult Americans are overweight, this is really worth thinking about. One of the more informative research studies in this line was that of Dr. Marvin Bierenbaum and his group from St. Vincent's Hospital in Montclair, New Jersey. They reported on their observations of a hundred men between thirty and fifty-four years of age after ten years of dietary treatment for their heart attacks. In the first five years, they found no difference in repeat heart attacks between half of the group who ate unsaturated oils and the other half who ate a saturated oil. There was also no difference in cholesterol and triglyceride levels. One reason for this might be that weight reduction was prescribed for all overweight members of either group, and their diet was restricted to 1200 calories.

Now comes the interesting part. Since there was no difference in morbidity between the groups, after five years a new control group was recruited. This consisted of 100 additional men, all of whom had also had a heart attack. However, there was one important difference: they averaged 24 pounds overweight and were not placed on weight-reducing, calorie-restricted diets. After five and ten years this control group had double the heart attacks and repeat heart attacks and fatalities. Clearly, the low-calorie diet and lower weight made a difference in mortality. By the way, there was no difference in cholesterol levels.

Recently, a whole town was studied to compare dietary habits with heart disease. Dr. A. B. Nichols and his group of researchers found that not 1 of the 110 food items evaluated, including cholesterol and fats, turned out to be significant in the 4,000 people in the study group. *The only thing that correlated with heart disease was excess body fat.* Blood cholesterol and triglycerides also were significantly related to overweight. The doctors concluded that the first thing to do in case of excess blood fats is to lose weight, not to cut out fats in the diet.

Nathan Pritikin, founder of the Longevity Research Institute, formerly of Santa Barbara but now relocated in Santa Monica, California, would dispute that interpretation, I am sure. His review of the scientific evidence has convinced him that a very low-fat, high complex carbohydrate diet is the only way to assure cardiovascular health. His applications of this principle have produced some very gratifying improvements in atherosclerotic heart disease, diabetes, obesity, hypertension, and arthritis, and he has been able to document these improvements with blood tests and X-ray arteriograms as well. In his writings he reminds us that Dr. Ancel Keys' Minnesota study confirms the initial Framingham results: the higher the blood cholesterol, the greater the risk of CHD. This was borne out also by Dr. C. C. Welch, who found by X-ray studies of arteries of 723 men under forty years old, half of whom had two main coronary arteries more than half closed, that the relationship of degree of artery closure to cholesterol level paralleled these statistics. In a similar vein, Dr. Irvine Page constructed a statistical table for prediction of artery closure based on age, blood cholesterol, and triglycerides. He then predicted with 98 percent accuracy which of 60 new patients would have closed arteries in the X rays.

Pritikin is particularly impressed by the incredible physical endurance of the Turahumara Indians of Mexico. A 48-hour-long game of kickball and a 500-mile run in five days have been described. These people subsist on 80 percent complex carbohydrate, mostly corn, peas, beans, squash, and other native flora. Animal protein is eaten only about once a month. Their cholesterol averages 100 to 130 milligrams, about half the average cholesterol level in this country. They also average 5 feet 7 inches and weigh 125 pounds. Degenerative diseases, such as CHD, diabetes, and arthritis, are virtually unknown.

Mr. Pritikin theorizes that fats, particularly essential fatty acids, are easily made into prostaglandins, which are triggers of platelet clumping. This can initiate clotting. In rabbits, fatal intravascular clotting follows almost immediately after intravenous injection of arachidonic acid, one of the essential fatty acids. Clearly an overdose of fat, particularly unsaturated fats, which contain more of these essential fatty acids, can be dangerous.

Finally, Pritikin quotes other research which indicates that fat intake is very definitely related to colon cancer. World Health Organization statistics show an almost one to one correlation: the higher the fat, the more bowel cancer. Dr. M. J. Hill, who performed this study, also found a hundredfold increase in anaerobic bacteria in the stools of such people. These are able to convert bile acids into carcinogens. Bacteria can also convert bile into estrogens, and this might stimulate tumor growth. Against this evidence, recall the previous chapter.

When we recall that Dr. Astrand found reduced endurance on high-fat diets and a three times greater endurance on a high-carbohydrate diet in cross-country skiers, along with the magnificent endurance of the Turahumara Indians, it is easy to understand why many joggers and runners swear by this diet.

On the other hand, not everyone is a runner or inclined to endurance exercise. Lots of people are convinced that civilization was designed to take us away from all that. I believe there must be a compromise between health needs and lifestyle requirements. The low-fat diet does seem to be advantageous in cases of diabetes and advanced atherosclerosis where there is no time to lose.

Let us not forget, however, that excellent results in degenerative diseases are available without going to the extreme that Mr. Pritikin recommends. No one yet knows whether mega-nutrition by itself, or in combination with dietary improvement, is as good as or better all around than this strict regimen.

What diet is right for you? If you are athletic and active and participating in endurance exercise, you will probably function better on the high-carbohydrate program. In a more sedentary person, often the result would be nervousness and irritability. And let us not forget that many people are unable to digest whole grains properly. Schizophrenics are often made worse by wheat. Cerebral allergy to wheat is also quite common and capable of inducing anxiety, depression, and paranoia!

Most important in rebuttal is the observation that Pritikin's diet therapy is without benefit of nutrient supplements. In view of the difficulty in obtaining fresh foods with their nutrient complement intact, this strikes me as foolhardy in the long term, especially since people who are ill require larger amounts of nutrients than usual. On the other hand, higher fat and protein also require larger amounts of nutrients. Carbohydrate molecules are smaller than fats and much smaller than proteins; it takes less energy to burn them in the body chemistry. We have already heard that increasing fat also increases the need for vitamin B_6 and magnesium up to tenfold. As for the clumping effect induced by blood fats, I am comforted by the anti-clumping effect of vitamins E and C and the extra protection conferred by a flush dose of niacin.

In short, despite the promise that Pritikin's work does hold, I am not convinced that it is necessary to abandon fat in food.

The fact remains that no one knows yet for certain what is the "one true way" to prevent CHD by dietary means. It may well be that there is no one true way, and each of us must find what works best for himself. Meanwhile, when your cholesterol and triglycerides are too high, it is good evidence that the body chemistry is being overloaded. It isn't healthy. But it isn't the triglycerides and cholesterol that do the harm. It's the strain on the system, the depletion of micronutrients by having to get rid of these excessive molecules and the physical interference with blood flow and oxygen exchange that occurs. Stay lean if you are at optimum weight. Lose weight if you are not.

Heart Rule No. 5: Avoid Sugar

I am referring *particularly* to refined sugar here: sucrose. Just as a case can be made for cholesterol or fat to be the culprit in CHD, there is an even stronger case for sugar. Dr. John Yudkin, you will recall, found that in all of the countries where Dr. Keys found that fat correlated with CHD, there was an even better correlation with increased sugar intake. One of Dr. Yudkin's most intriguing studies compared a group of men who had had heart attacks to a healthy control group. The sugar consumption averaged almost twice as much in the heart attack group, 140 pounds per year, compared to an average of 80 pounds per year in the healthy group. Yudkin concluded that a daily intake of 4 ounces of sugar carries a five times greater risk of heart disease than 2 ounces of sugar would.

The numerous other reasons for cutting back on sugar will be thoroughly discussed in Chapter 7.

Heart Rule No. 6: Get the Right Potassium Balance

It may surprise you to learn that salt, which you have always been told is bad for you, is actually good—in its place. Salt has been blamed as the leading cause of high blood pressure, but that turns out not to be true. All studies indicate that potassium correlates more truly to blood pressure regulation than does salt. Hormonal regulation of blood pressure does most of the real controlling. Salt is controlled by appetite, regulated by taste and by certain receptors in the brain that constantly monitor the blood.

Salt your food according to your needs: energy and taste. If you are salting your food and do not have high blood pressure, there is probably no need to reduce your salt intake. If you do have a tendency to high blood pressure but also a craving for salt, ask your doctor about taking supplementary potassium. (Use a potassium salt or mixed sodium-potassium combination.)

Salt hasn't much to do with elevated blood pressure at all, especially in the moderate amounts apparently eaten in the United States. One study, in fact, found that in the relationship between salt preference, salt threshold, and weight relative to blood pressure in 4,800 school children, it was body weight that had a significant impact on blood pressure and not either of the salt influences.

Although there are still a great many scientists and physicians who adhere to the salt theory of elevated blood pressure, it should be noted that most of the evidence indicating that salt is a contributary factor indicates only that it contributes when taken in *extremely* large amounts, amounts which no person would ingest voluntarily without some kind of pathological compulsion for salt.

Although mankind's appetite for salt is conditioned, studies show that the salt/hypertension correlation varies greatly from population to population: in the United States we have no great craving for huge amounts. The usual daily intake in this country is about seven grams. A lunch including biscuits and canned soup gives you about 3.5 grams; a TV dinner with salad and dressing in the evening will add 4 more grams, and there you have it. Without even sprinkling table salt on anything, one can achieve the seven-gram average quite easily.

Are you low, average, or high in your salt intake? Roland L. Weinsier of the U.S. Air Force School of Aerospace Medicine, after studying 1,246 adults, classified them as *low* when they never add salt to their food; *average* when they add salt only after tasting; and *high* when they customarily add salt to food before tasting it. Hence, if you never add salt to food, or only add it when you've tasted the food first, you probably have no reason to cut down your salt intake for fear of elevating your blood pressure.

However, evidence strongly indicates that, at the same time, you should be paying attention to your potassium level, for potassium seems to counteract whatever hypertensive effects salt *might* have on your system. In other words, a low potassium level is a better indicator of potential high blood pressure problems, and an elevated potassium intake is a better *modifier* of hypertension than is salt abstinence.

Both salt (sodium) and potassium are essential nutrients for sustaining life, but evidence shows potassium appears to be required in larger amounts than heretofore believed.

Potassium chloride, when added to sodium chloride (table salt), produces a good sodium/potassium balance that is acceptable as regular table salt. Since the evidence indicates that potassium counteracts the possible hypertensive effects of high doses of sodium, this mixture would seem to be a good idea for anyone considering reducing salt intake for cardiac health reasons. (There are commercial preparations available that balance potassium and sodium for kitchen use, as mentioned earlier.)

W. Gordon Walker, M.D., Professor of Medicine and Director of the Kidney and Hypertension Division of Johns Hopkins, found that a statistical analysis of 574 patients showed no correlation between sodium and either blood pressure, aldosterone, or plasma-renin activity, but that low potassium *was significantly correlated with all three.* And at the same university, George D. Miller, M.D., of the School of Hygiene and Public Health, studied 2,500 blacks and whites, finding that high levels of dietary potassium can protect against hypertension. He told the American Heart Association that "potassium almost makes sodium a moot entity."

So, recent evidence strongly suggests that increased potassium can offset the hypertensive effects of salt and that your salt intake in the first place needn't be the source of worry, unless you're an above-average salt consumer. This means you should eat sunflower seeds (the best source of potassium), bananas, fresh vegetables, orange juice, beans, nuts, molasses and meats, and above all *avoid processed foods!*

Heart Rule No. 7: Check Your HDL (High-Density Lipoproteins)

At your next checkup, have your doctor order a test of high-density lipoproteins (HDL), a newly recognized blood factor that has a protective effect against cholesterol deposits and CHD. These are "healthy" fats, containing a high ratio of protein to fat (lipoprotein is literally "fat protein"), necessary to transport cholesterol and other substances safely and solubly to the blood vessels. It is now known that there is an inverse relationship between the level of HDL in your blood and the risk of atherosclerotic heart disease. That is, the higher the level of HDL, the lower the risk. The Framingham study showed that patients who suffered heart attacks did not necessarily have high blood-fat levels, but almost always showed low levels of high-density lipoproteins. Subsequent studies have corroborated this relationship. Recent reductions in the rate of heart disease in the United States can be explained by the increase in aerobic exercise, which elevates HDL, and the growing use of vitamins C and E. When other important micronutrients, such as magnesium, zinc, copper, selenium and chromium, are better appreciated and more widely used, the epidemic will decline further. As more physicians and patients alike recognize the scientific validity of mega-nutrition and change their diets accordingly, the epidemic of CHD will finally end.

Heart Rule No. 8: Train Yourself in the Relaxation Response

Relaxation is the elusive butterfly of cardiac health. We all know what it is; we can easily identify it when we see it; and indeed we admire it and strive to emulate it.

However, the biological individuality that is continually emphasized throughout this book also applies to our mental state. That is, just as one person requires 2 grams of vitamin C per day for optimal health and another can tolerate 8 or 12 grams per day, so it is with our ability to relax and take things in stride. Many of us can simply sit back, take a deep breath and reduce anxiety. Others—the so-called Type A personalities—require more structured and definite regimens to achieve the same result.

Everyone should learn a technique to achieve the "relaxation response." Whether it's signing up for a class in Transcendental Meditation, or learning a system of self-hypnosis, or simply training oneself to respond to one's own "mantra," or "word," we are all capable of acquiring a self-relaxation stimulant. It's beyond the scope of this book to delve into the complexities of automatic methods of relaxation. I recommend that anyone who feels tense, anxious, or vaguely "uptight" should go to the library and examine the battery of books purporting to lead to inner peace. If something appeals to you, take it up with your physician or a licensed counselor—or listen to what has worked for your friends.

These eight guidelines for maintaining a healthy heart aren't just my opinions but rather established scientific correlations and cause-and-effect relationships. I have left out two possible precursors of heart disease—chlorinated water and homogenized milk, discussed in the previous chapter—because they are still subject to debate on scientific grounds. I happen to believe, on the strength of the evidence to date, that they are harmful. I leave it up to you to take the same precautions I do: (1) let the chlorine vaporize by storing tap water in an open container for a few hours, and (2) avoid homogenized milk or heat to near boiling, 92°C., for a few seconds.

There are some things we have no control over in heart disease risk, such as genetics. If both your parents are past the age of seventy-five, you're in luck: you'll probably live to that age without heart disease, too. Certainly, following these guidelines can only vastly improve your heart's health and decrease your likelihood of CHD problems.

The Nutrition Prescription for a Healthy Heart

- Eat a range of foods that give you trace minerals and such key vitamins as C, E, and B_6
- Do some exercise every day, vigorously on a regular basis—good diet and exercise raise your vital HDL cholesterol
- Don't smoke, avoid refined sugar, and balance your salt intake with ample potassium
- Maintain your optimal weight
- Support your good eating habits with relaxation techniques

6
Cancer: Your Body Is the Answer

Why is it that cancer is such a terrifying and perplexing subject? We avoid its very name, preferring a euphemism like "malignancy" or "the big C." Some astrologers have substituted "Moon" for it among the astrological signs. Susan Sontag deplores, in her book *Illness As Metaphor*, the use of the word as a metaphor for any horrible aberration in society or politics. Cancer appears to be a sinister, uncontrollable enemy simply because it is *multifarious*—and our paradigm of medical treatment is that for each disease there is a single knowable cause and a single best therapy.

It's time to face cancer squarely for what it is: not necessarily any worse and often quite a bit better than the other major "killer" diseases. Consider these facts about it:

- Cancer usually gives an early warning, sometimes nothing more than fatigue or mood depression rather than physical pain or malfunction.
- Cancer often waits a good long time before putting in a physical appearance—20 or 30 years of delay isn't unusual—thereby giving us ample time to do something to build up our resistance and prevent its spread.
- When cancer does appear it often looks no more vicious than a

bump on the skin or a sore that won't heal properly. In fact, more than a fourth of all cancers are so hidden that they're not diagnosed at all—though half of these are fatal.
• Many cancers are rightly considered curable, in the sense that remissions of five years or longer are consistently observed.

At the same time, some ominous signs of our inability to control the major cancers persist, and for a variety of illogical reasons a cancer phobia continues to be promulgated, much to the ultimate detriment of an uninformed public. I frequently see patients who are unwilling to face the warning signs of cancer because of their fear of current cancer therapy. They become fatalistic without reason or, in the other extreme, they accede all to readily to massive surgery or chemotherapy and thus prove what they most fear. The central theme of this chapter is that there's plenty you can do about cancer of any kind, if you can overcome your own fears and the artificial restraints of conventional wisdom about cancer therapy.

It's the Law: I Can't Make a Nutrition Prescription for Cancer

Largely as a legacy of the history of laetrile in California, where I practice, it's against the law for me to prescribe nutritional therapy for cancer of any kind. To put the matter bluntly, I'm forbidden to practice what I preach.

To see how limiting this sort of law is, consider the case of Alice M., who had it within her means to do anything she wished to fight her cancer. She came to me for nutritional advice, yet it was hard to believe she was desperately ill. Attractive, younger in appearance than her forty years, well-dressed, she was also intelligent and down to earth in her questions. She had just relapsed after eight years of remission from breast cancer. Now she wanted to know if anything further could be done. Money was no object: she was the sole heir to a Texas-size fortune and could fly anywhere in the world in her own jet.

Hers was a story of self-reliance and good luck—or she wouldn't have made it through the surgery and radiation therapy eight years before. In addition to her excellent treatment she had started herself on a natural-foods diet and vitamin regimen. Everything had gone well until eight months before her visit to me. Then, unexpectedly, her husband died. He had been the healthy one, with a comfortable lifestyle and not a care in the world. But she had taken the vitamins—because she was the sick one.

Alice knew enough about cancer to realize that stress and depression can trigger a recurrence, but she was unable to contain her grief. She had had the rare good fortune of a happy and satisfying marriage. Childless, she and her husband had been inseparable. So the first few weeks of loneliness took a lot out of her. In spite of her excellent dietary precautions, within a month she discovered a nodule—a sign of metastasis, or spread—of the cancer. At once she consulted leading cancer specialists in her local area and in New York. She received the latest anti-cancer drugs: Cytoxan, 5-fluoro-uracil, Adriamycin, Leukeran, and BCG vaccine. Yet this advanced form of chemotherapy only left her weak and depressed, while the nodules of cancer cells remained painfully evident in the area of her mastectomy. She was afraid she was going to die from this relapse.

On examination she seemed healthy enough except for the bumps in her chest and a swollen arm due to the removal of lymphatics in the original surgery. But computer analysis of her diet turned up serious deficiencies: lack of vitamin A and zinc, known to weaken the immune system by reducing the formation of antibodies; lack of the B vitamin folic acid, hindering the formation of nucleic acids in cell repair; and low levels of the protein amino acid methionine, further reducing the ability to produce antibodies. To indicate the value of nutritional testing even in cases less life-threatening than this, here is a rundown of additional *laboratory* findings:

- Her folic acid proved to be borderline low, 5 nanograms (ng) compared to a normal range of 5–20 nanograms.
- Similarly, her vitamin B_{12}, also necessary in cell regeneration, or healing, was only 295 picograms (pg) compared to a normal range of 200–900.
- Her white blood cells, which target and destroy cancer cells as well as other harmful substances, were also reduced to about half the normal *low* amount—not surprising in view of her recent treatment by chemotherapy, which destroys some healthy cells along with cancer cells—yet it was two months since the last treatment and her count was 2,700 compared to a normal range of 5,000 to 10,000.
- Hair analysis showed very low levels of magnesium, manganese, and copper—all essential in the energy-producing and tissue-repair functions of the body.

• Her unusually high level of fluoride, 9.3 parts per million as opposed to a normal level of less than 1 part per million, presumably the result of such medications as 5-fluoro-uracil, suggested further depletion of minerals, since fluoride is highly toxic and can inactivate such minerals as magnesium by forming insoluble substances.

Most alarming of all the laboratory findings was the report of low blood serum vitamin A—half the normal minimum. I explained to Alice that vitamin A had been known to be protective against some forms of cancer since the 1920s and that more recent experience indicated that vitamin A is particularly important in breast cancer. Yet I had to advise her that I could make no claims or offer direct counsel about treating her cancer with vitamin supplements. In my state the nutritional treatment of cancer is illegal.

All I could do was prescribe a *general* nutritional program, however, making sure it included the critical vitamins and minerals shown to be low in the laboratory, hair, and dietary analyses above. I could discuss the promising research of Linus Pauling and Ewan Cameron in treating cancer with megadoses of ascorbate, vitamin C, and I could prescribe extra vitamin E and selenium for her general health. I could encourage her to avoid overloading her system with proteins, especially from animal sources, as these are known to carry numerous microorganisms associated with tumors. I could also advise her to increase her intake of methionine through vegetable sources, such as beans, legumes, and whole grains—merely to build up her general resistance. *But I could not prescribe nutritionally to the best of my ability because of the law.* And in my caution I'm afraid I was less convincing in my general nutritional advice than I might otherwise have been.

Six months later she flew back to San Francisco, more desperate than ever. She explained that she hadn't taken any nutrient supplements for fear of "jarring" her metabolism. Somehow she had gotten the idea from her cancer specialists that vitamins might do her harm; she gave up even the vitamins she had been taking for years. Instead she agreed to one course of chemotherapy. It was certainly not comforting to be told by one of her doctors that "if only one more inch of lymph nodes had been irradiated" the previous summer, the cancer would have been contained.

It was clear Alice didn't know what to believe. My hands were tied. She bade me farewell and headed her jet for Lourdes. Three months later she was dead.

The research information on vitamin A that I was unable to bring to Alice's attention goes back to work in Germany since 1966. Dr. Hans Hoefer-Janker has pioneered in megadose vitamin A therapy in amounts up to 1,000 times the RDA of 5,000 units a day. You are probably aware of the fact that extremely high doses of A can be toxic—deaths and liver damage have been reported from eating large amounts of polar bear liver, which is exceptionally rich in this vitamin. The European treatment is possible only because of a special emulsion of vitamin A, which by-passes the liver. In 1976 Dr. Frank Chytil of Vanderbilt University reported that tumors containing the vitamin A-binding protein mentioned above were found to be curable with large doses of the vitamin. And the emulsion form of vitamin A has been especially successful in conjunction with proteolytic enzymes and certain anticancer drugs. As a result of these findings, the National Cancer Institute has recently initiated studies of the vitamin A emulsion derivative. This form of vitamin A, however, is not available for general use in the United States.

A New Look at Cancer Therapy—Even Laetrile

Are cancer patients, like Alice, the victims of an overly restricted approach to therapy? I feel strongly that they are. But the underlying problem of current work in oncology—the study of cancer—can be summarized in one phrase: the patient has been treated as a passive specimen. As Pauling and Cameron write, "There is increasing awareness among oncologists that, irrespective of the definitive anti-cancer treatment employed, the progress and eventual outcome of any cancer illness depend upon the inherent natural resistance of the patient."

Perhaps if physicians talked more about increasing patients' inherent natural resistance, and less in terms of *treating* them with nutrition, we would not be threatened by the type of law that prohibits laetrile. The two things, of course, come down to the same prescription: improving the patient's intake of essential vitamins and minerals, from foods or supplements.

What are the results of the three major cancer therapies in vogue since the Second World War—radiation, surgery, and chemotherapy? In many cases, spectacular successes. As Pauling and Cameron insist, "In the present state of our knowledge, clinicians have a clear duty to remove the main tumor cell mass if at all possible" by any or all of these methods. Nevertheless, as D. S. Greenberg concluded in a survey in the *New England Journal of Medicine* in 1975, the survival rates for the *majority* of cancer patients have shown no improvement over the 25 years in which cytotoxic (cell-killing) chemotherapy has been more and more aggressively employed.

In 25 years, in the majority of cancers, no improvement. Why? Why has the "cancer establishment," as the well-funded oncology centers are often referred to, poured its money into the search for more and stronger drugs, and fiercely resisted nutritional approaches? Well, medicine has always been a cautious enterprise.

There are ten major factors in the development of cancer that we can pinpoint with any certainty at all.

- Smoking
- Occupational pollutants
- Excessive sunlight and background radiation
- Pesticides/additives/hormones in foods
- Water pollution (including chlorine and fluoride)
- Undernutrition (including lack of fiber)
- Air pollution
- Alcohol
- Certain medical drugs
- Stressful moods

All of these are carcinogenic (cancer-causing) substances or conditions. Various theorists have related all of these causes to stress, but it seems more helpful to know the more immediate causes. We also have identified thousands of epidemiological—demographic—factors, which may or may not give us a clue to a proximate cause but do not give us any information which suggests preventive measures. For example, we know that small-breasted women have 30 times greater risk of breast cancer than large-breasted women. Thus, we do know that hormonal and hereditary factors must be considered. Researchers have developed special breeds of laboratory animals that develop spontaneous cancers in predictable numbers at predictable times. This possibility has greatly enhanced our research capabilities. But if you are interested in your own health you are more likely concerned with what you can do at this time to avoid the known carcinogens.

Cancer cells, no matter what tissue or organ they inhabit, seem to break the rules of normal cell behavior. Their "contact inhibitors" fail, they continue to divide, and so they grow uncontrollably. They act like parasites, burning valuable fuels and producing toxic waste products that crowd out and poison normal cells in their vicinity. Why do carcinogens start cells on this binge of destruction?

When dogs inhale smoke in the laboratory, they contract lung cancer. When tobacco tars are applied to the skin of laboratory animals, they get skin cancer. Smoking is known to be responsible for the great increase in lung cancer in this century, and now that women have been smoking as much as men the lung cancer rate is the same for both. Cigarette smoke will cause cancer in anyone in time; it simply takes longer for some than for others. We know all this not only by examining statistics but by noting obvious damage to the lungs of smokers. The evidence is very convincing, except perhaps to smokers and tobacco companies.

The search for a "safer" cigarette is a cruel euphemism in the light of the fact that smokers are known to inhale smoke especially for the effects of nicotine. Chain smokers over the age of 55 have 80 times greater risk of lung cancer than nonsmokers. Only 1 nonsmoker in 3,300 dies of lung cancer, while 1 in 40 chain smokers do. Two-pack-a-day smokers age forty give up eight years of their life expectancy.

I mention this leading cancer-causing substance not as a brief message from the American Cancer Society, but as a primary example of a new approach that's necessary in cancer prevention. We have all heard these statistics and more, yet smoking continues unabated and is even promoted to some extent by the federal government by its subsidies to the tobacco industry. Why? I think it's because the dedicated and habituated smoker clutches at the few straws of evidence that shift the blame to "tars" that are supposedly under continual reduction in cigarettes. What people should be told is that cigarette smoke also contains carbon monoxide, cadmium, arsenic, and lead. These poisons not only reduce the body's general resistance to cancer but can also damage blood vessels and cause heart disease. In effect, I would like to see the emphasis on carcinogens shifted to the general weakening of the body's defenses that they cause, and not confined to a few specific maladies. *Cigarette smokers live shorter lives, and they die more painful and prolonged deaths.*

Carcinogens Don't Exist in the Abstract

The human body is a surprisingly tough organism. As a doctor I'm less surprised by the high mortality rates of smokers than by the fact that some heavy smokers apparently show few ill effects from the poisons they inhale. The body has immense resources; it can tolerate poisons to some degree if, on balance, worse poisons are thereby avoided. A case in point is the subject of food additives.

It's quite true that some food-coloring agents, preservatives, and other additives have been identified as carcinogens. This fact, unfortunately, isn't balanced by the knowledge that many of the same additives contribute more to health in other ways than they detract from health as carcinogens. No matter what we put into our bodies, it involves a trade-off of risks against benefits. Nothing is 100 percent good, nothing 100 percent bad. Put this way, the matter seems obvious; yet we have a law, the Delaney Clause of 1958, which forbids the marketing of a product shown to have any carcinogenic properties at all—regardless of its good points. And there are all sorts of consumer advocates to whom the word "additive" is anathema. It's difficult to know which way to turn, be one a scientist or simply a caring homemaker.

- Is salt bad because it's associated with hypertension in some people, or do we need it for the iodine?
- Do we need extra iodine, or do we get ample amounts in seafood?
- Should we banish all fat, including fish oils, or do we need the prostacyclins in fish to help prevent clotting?
- Should we eat only egg whites, because of the danger of dietary cholesterol, or do we need all the nutrients of the yolk to help prevent damage to blood vessels?

I've touched on these issues already. What about a carcinogen, however, like nitrates? Of the 3,000 or more chemicals currently being added to processed foods, carcinogens like cyclamate and nitrates have been heavily publicized. A case can perhaps be made for an artificial sweetener, like saccharine, because of the dangers of the sugar it replaces. Do nitrates deserve the notoriety they have received?

Nitrates are added to ham, sausage, bacon, and hot dogs to preserve flavor and add an appealing red color. But as preservatives they perform the far more important function of preventing the growth of a poisonous bacterium, *Clostridium botulinum,* which, as the name suggests, causes botulism. This is the deadliest poison known to man. The minor risk of cancer from nitrates in bacon—projected from animal experiments involving huge amounts of nitrate—is, in my opinion, a reasonable trade-off against the major risk of death from botulism.

Better yet, we can also protect ourselves from the minor risk in the bargain! In all the wailing and moaning about nitrates, there has been little mention of the fact that we have an effective antidote to the possible carcinogenic properties of nitrates. It's vitamin C—here, as in many other cases, a substance of surprising powers. Ascorbate has been shown to prevent harmless nitrate from converting to the *toxic* element nitrosamine when nitrate is exposed to the acid digestion process in the stomach and small intestine. Look at the labels of packaged meats and you'll find a number of them indicating ascorbate has been added—precisely for this reason.

A similar example of dietary protection against additives suspected of being carcinogens is the case of certain yellow dyes. Food dyes have been in the news in recent years, but as long ago as 1923 it was known that dyes used in breads and margarines were capable of producing bladder cancer in mice. At the same time it was observed that animals treated with vitamin A did not develop the same cancer. Why was the observation overlooked for all these years?

As I've mentioned in the case of Alice M., vitamin A has recently created quite a stir among oncologists because of success with it in European cancer centers and current testing by the National Cancer Institute. Many think of it as a great new discovery—yet the laboratory and experimental indications have been known for more than 50 years!

My point about carcinogens is this: the word itself has become another scare word, like "cancer." We need to face the fact of carcinogens realistically. Sometimes we can accept them as the lesser of two risks, and even then we may be able to protect ourselves against the risk. Now, if nutrition in the form of vitamin supplementation can offer protection against cancer-causing agents, how about nutrition in cancer *treatment?*

Fighting the Ghost of Quackery

To some, laetrile means hope in an impossible situation; to others, the struggle of rights against bureaucracy; to still others, perhaps the majority, it means quackery. As of this writing, some 13 states have legalized laetrile treatment—over the objection of organized medicine, the cancer institutes, and federal agencies. The political lobbying for this drug, or vitamin, or whatever you want to call it, is often pictured as tainted with avaricious promoters, just as the medical lobby for it was pictured as peopled with unscrupulous doctors. I bring up laetrile at this point because in the background of any discussion of the utility of nutrition against cancer is the specter of this highly publicized product, once banned in almost every country except Germany and Mexico and declared useless by the most respected research center in the United States.

If laetrile had proved to be the worthless hoax it has been branded, vitamin and mineral therapy against cancer could still stand, of course, on its own merits. Yet it now appears that even laetrile may prove to have some value in a *carefully monitored, complete program*. The subject is a controversial one and there is a danger of becoming a zealot on either side of the issue. I will present the most recent findings with the understanding that these are tentative and should not be used to condemn the conscientious work of those who have investigated it in the past.

Laetrile is a substance naturally occurring in apricot pits and bitter almonds. It is also dubbed amygdalin and, more recently, vitamin B_{17} by Dr. Ernest Krebs, who first researched it and became its ardent promoter. (It's worth noting that Dr. Krebs and his father had sound reputations in medical research before their controversial work on laetrile.) In California, where it was first used clinically on cancer patients, laetrile had a checkered career for almost two decades before it vaulted to national prominence on the strength of a tentatively favorable report, on a study by Dr. Kanematsu Sugiura from the Sloan-Kettering Institute for Cancer Research. A violent reaction ensued, in which the promising tests were repeated and other researchers began to bear down heavily on the claims of laetrile's promoters. Their conclusion was that laetrile was at best a placebo and at worst a menace to gullible patients who might otherwise seek out conventional therapy. The FDA stepped up its enforcement of its ban of this drug, doctors using laetrile were brought to court in California and elsewhere, and patients flocked in ever-greater numbers across the border to laetrile clinics.

In their fervor to protect cancer victims from themselves, the regulators took little notice of the fact that conventional treatment has unique perils of its own. Dr. Hardin Jones has raised the question of whether conventional cancer treatment might not make some cases worse. Surely the adverse effects are sufficient so that some regard the treatment as worse than the disease! Conventional treatment has been effective in many cases, to be sure, but the appeal of laetrile was mainly to hopeless cases or to patients who had reason to fear the substantial side effects of cytotoxic drugs and radiation.

Even though *The New York Times* argued in favor of allowing patients to choose laetrile, medical authorities generally considered the matter a closed case and spoke in terms of laetrile victims being preyed upon by sharp promoters. Then along came Dr. Harold Manner, chairman of the biology department at Loyola University in Chicago. In 1978 he caused a sensation at the National Health Federation meeting in Chicago by reporting that he had reached a 90 percent cure rate of spontaneous breast cancer in mice, and improvement in the rest, with laetrile. As recommended by laetrile clinics, Dr. Manner's treatment included a total nutritional supplemental program—in this case vitamin A emulsion and proteolytic enzymes. The cancer cells were killed and turned into a pus that was easily excreted. Dr. Manner's work was immediately criticized as being based on gross observations rather than microscopic proof of tumor remissions; he rebutted that the disappearance of tumors is usually accepted as proof enough. Although as of this writing his experiments haven't been duplicated in other laboratories, there can be little doubt that such startling and unequivocal results have some validity. His is the first clear-cut signal that in spite of a dubious history laetrile is a factor to consider in cancer treatment.

Why, then, were previous experiments negative or at best marginal with respect to laetrile's efficacy? One explanation is that *transplanted* tumors were generally used in all of the previous laboratory experiments. These tumors are developed in laboratory animals by grinding up cancer cells and injecting them at the spot where the cancer is desired. The tumors probably are the result of overwhelming infection by virus particles that interact with nucleic acids of the host, the animal. *Spontaneous* cancers, on the other hand, represent a weakness in the immune or repair system of the cell, perhaps because of a vitamin or mineral deficiency resulting from a hereditary inability to absorb or transport essential nutrients. Cells then become susceptible to such carcinogens as free radicals. Unlike his predecessors, Dr. Manner selected his mice from a strain known to develop cancer.

How laetrile works, when and if it does, had also defied convincing explanation until Dr. Manner's studies. That it was a vitamin was ridiculed on the grounds that it had no known function in the body. Dr. Ernest Krebs had theorized that the laetrile molecule releases cyanide into the cancer cells it enters and that an enzyme present only in normal cells prevents laetrile from readily breaking down into cyanide. Dr. Manner studied the tissues of his experimental animals and found that cyanide was indeed concentrated in the tumor tissues. As the dosage of laetrile was increased, larger amounts of harmless thiocyaniate were excreted in the urine. Thus the by-product of cyanide was being re-

moved, and animals on large doses of laetrile actually appeared healthier than the control animals.

A less direct approach to determining the efficacy of laetrile came
recently as a result of a public outcry over its prohibition. The National
Cancer Institute was asked to evaluate as many valid and acceptable
laetrile case histories—of human subjects, of course—as they could find
and compare them with case histories of those treated with conventional
methods. Without being told which type of treatment was given, a panel
of scientists reviewed the cases and found that the *use of laetrile alone
resulted in a cure rate comparable to the others:* 4 out of 22 laetrile patients were considered cured—an 18 percent rate.

Surprised officials have now approved formal testing under the auspi-
ces of the NCI. The pendulum has finally swung, even for lowly laetrile.

Many drugs are efficacious, of course, without being safe, but efficacy
is far more difficult to show. For a time, the FDA rejected laetrile as
also being unsafe. Taking laetrile by injection overcomes the problem of
overdosing, another reason why laetrile should be given by a physician.
The nutritional program recommended by laetrile proponents also has
preventive elements, though it is intended primarily to enhance the
effect of laetrile. The proteolytic enzymes I have referred to are
believed by Dr. Manner to help strip away proteins that cover cancer
cells and thus make it easier for the body's immune system to target
them. In spite of all the adverse publicity about laetrile from a handful
of cases of overdose, when properly administered there is evidence that
it is both safe and effective enough to warrant consideration in a complete therapeutic program.

The Case for Nutrition against Cancer

There is always a considerable time lag between the scientific validation
of a medical treatment and its acceptance by the general public, by state
legislatures, and by federal agencies. The bias against nutrition is especially deep-seated, particularly in the case of cancer treatment and prevention. Dr. Stanley Dudrick, a pioneer in intravenous feeding in the
treatment of cancer, notes, "Up until 1972 there was a taboo that said
if you fed a cancer patient you would accelerate the growth of the
tumor. We've found that to be untrue."

The feed-the-tumor fallacy wasn't put to rest until research at M. D.
Anderson Hospital in Houston in 1977 showed conclusively that intravenous feeding of a total complement of nutrients was beneficial to pa-

tients already undergoing standard treatment. Patients were able to tolerate chemotherapy to a greater degree and experienced fewer side effects. A drastic use of nutrients, in what has come to be called a "rescue" treatment, was tried successfully at about the same time at the Sloan-Kettering Institute in New York City. Remissions in extreme cases were obtained by using very high doses of anti-cancer drugs and then administering vitamins to pull the patients back from the imminent death that could be expected from the chemotherapy.

Another step toward an orthomedical treatment of cancer is in the growing use of folic acid in conjunction with certain cancer drugs. Folic acid aids in regenerating cells, and this action is blocked by drugs like Methotrexate. When such cancer drugs are used, supplemental folic acid compensates for their antagonistic effect against the body's existing level of this member of the B vitamin complex.

The tentative results of such nutrients as laetrile, vitamin A, folic acid, and a general supplemental program of vitamins and minerals are significant for cancer treatment, but perhaps not as important in the long run as the apparent success of nutrients of many kinds in strengthening the body's immune system. Several West Coast names stand out in this work: Dr. Virginia Livingston in San Diego; Dr. Benjamin V. Siegel in Portland; and Drs. Linus Pauling and Ewan Cameron in Menlo Park. For years, against the background of conventional emphasis on chemotherapy, Dr. Livingston has persevered in researching immunological techniques. Dr. Siegel more recently has been studying the connection between anti-viral activities in the body and vitamin C. And Drs. Pauling and Cameron have almost singlehandedly undertaken clinical studies of vitamin C in the treatment of advanced cancers.

At her San Diego treatment center, Dr. Livingston identified, as long ago as 1947, a specific virus present in all cancers—the microbe *Progenitor Cryptocides*. The medical establishment at first rejected her breakthrough discovery and cut off her research funds, looking askance at the dietary, orthomolecular therapy she employed to build up the body's immune system against this virus. *P. Cryptocides* has the characteristic of changing from a rod-shaped bacterium into a more primitive acellular virus, much like a tubercle bacillus. Viral activity remains after the bacterial cell wall has broken down; the viral fragment combines with the nucleic acids, the DNA of body cells. The growth and activity of the cells is accordingly changed to a cancerous state. This brief and simplistic description isn't intended to convince the scientist *or* the layperson; the point is that Dr. Livingston found a rationale in the relationship between *Cryptocides* and the tubercle bacillus to explain the successful use of the BCG vaccine—using tubercle bacilli to develop immunity—in the treatment of some cancers. (BCG has been used successfully for many years, without general agreement on the mechanism involved.) Dr. Livingston, however, went one step further.

Working with *Cryptocides* strains taken from cancerous animals, she developed vaccines to support the immune system. Eventually, her work led to the development of vaccines specific to individual cancer patients from strains taken from their own bodies. Though she has now gained a respected international following, Dr. Livingston is careful to qualify her work: she isn't curing cancer, but helping the body build up its own immunity.

To support her therapy, Dr. Livingston provides her patients with a controversial nutritional regimen—and this is what the medical establishment seems to have difficulty accepting. Because she found that meat and dairy products are heavily infested with *Cryptocides* organisms, she recommends minimizing those foods in the diet. She suspects that many animals slaughtered for human consumption have cancer themselves, and some of the meat finds its way into our diet. Exposure to infected organisms theoretically could stimulate the body to produce protective antibodies. Against this possibility Dr. Livingston argues that a body depleted in nutrients might be unable to rise to the challenge. And since most meats and fowl are aged (beef becomes tender through bacteriological action), organisms are likely to have multiplied prodigiously before reaching our tables. For all of these reasons, Dr. Livingston includes antibiotics along with the vitamins, minerals, and vaccine in her therapy program.

Enhancing the body's immune system is also the cancer specialty of Professor Siegel of the University of Oregon Health Sciences Center in Portland. Dr. Siegel's work focuses on a new direction in research, the ability of the body to produce an anti-viral substance called *interferon*. In synthetic form, this substance is still quite expensive and available only in small amounts for research. The evidence seems to indicate, however, that vitamin C induces the body to produce interferon. One study of mice infected with a leukemia virus, for example, showed that those given large amounts of ascorbate produced twice the interferon of those not receiving vitamin C.

Dr. Siegel has also been able to explain the mechanism by which interferon works: it enhances the activity of macrophages, large white blood cells that ingest and destroy the harmful cells of a virus or cancer. Vitamin C also activates white cells from the thymus gland, T-cells. Virus or cancer cells contact T-cells, which become sensitized and then release hormones (lymphokines) that in turn activate more macrophages. Thus relatively few T-cells can lead to the stimulation of large numbers of macrophages. In broad terms this is the picture of how the body's immune system works. The enveloping and digesting of "enemy" cells (viral or cancer) is called phagocytosis; T-cells may be thought of as a sort of vigilante squad patrolling the body and prepared to signal phagocytosis to start.

In confirming Linus Pauling's tentative explanation of how ascorbate assists the immune system against cancer, Dr. Siegel has made a crucial contribution to the whole case for vitamin C in megadoses. "The more experiments I do," he says, "the more vitamin C I take."

At the moment, the Siegel paradigm for the activity of ascorbate on the immune system is convincing enough. Clinical results are even more reassuring. Drs. Pauling and Cameron have recently provided the most compelling evidence based on the results of several years of studies of treatment of terminal cancer patients at the Vale of Leven Hospital in Scotland.

In 1966 Dr. Cameron proposed that sufficient levels of ascorbate might render the protective mechanisms of the body powerful enough to achieve control of cancer, or retard it. Every cell in the body is held together by an intricate intracellular cement made up of collagen fibrils, called "ground substance." The fibrils form a tough, fibrous protein material that holds cells in place within the tissues. The natural enemy of the fibrils are certain enzymes, hyaluronidase and collagenase: these are liberated by malignant tumors and attack the fibrils and tissues around the tumor. Thus the cancer cell invades surrounding tissues, gaining fuel and multiplying. Cameron contended that ascorbate builds the resistance of collagen fibrils to attack by hyaluronidase and collagenase.

Ten years later he was able to report, in the *Proceedings of the National Academy of Sciences,* that the use of supplemental ascorbate prolonged the life expectancy of cancer patients as much as eight times. Linus Pauling was now collaborating with him, bringing valuable statistical methodology to bear on the difficult problem of accounting for numerous variables from one patient to the next. For each of 100 "untreatable" patients volunteering to take vitamin C in megadoses, ten untreatable controls were selected from the same hospital, matched as closely as possible by sex, age, primary tumor type, and clinical status. As of mid-1976, since the start of treatment the ascorbate-treated patients had lived an average of more than four times longer than the matched controls. By late 1979, the ratio was approaching an average of six to one.

Recently, working together at the Linus Pauling Institute in Menlo Park, California, Cameron and Pauling have elaborated on the mechanism they believe responsible for the effectiveness of ascorbate against cancer. Among the factors involved, they assert, are "integrity of the intercellular matrix, the passive role of collagen in strengthening the matrix and its active role in the protective encapsulation of tumors, the control of invasive enzymes, hormone balance, immunocompetence, and phagocytosis." Their conclusion: "Many, if not all, of the factors involved in host resistance to neoplasia (tumor growth) are significantly dependent upon the availability of ascorbate." Should vitamin C treatment be standard procedure in cancer treatment? They put the case directly: "Supplemental ascorbate is of some value to all cancer patients and can be of dramatic benefit to a fortunate few."

Has the evidence supporting nutritional approaches to cancer impressed the "cancer establishment," as its opponents call it? After some 30 years of neglect, it appears that the well-funded cancer organizations in this country are beginning to listen to the claims of the nutritionists. In mid-1979, the National Cancer Institute committed itself to a significant budget increase for research into nutrition. Gio Gori of the NCI was named editor of a journal that made its appearance in late 1979. Its title: *Nutrition and Cancer*.

How Nutrition Protects against Carcinogens

At the beginning of this chapter I referred to the ten major causes of cancer and indicated some of the simplest ways in which vitamins and minerals guard against certain carcinogens. Let's now turn to this subject in greater detail. Very often when we understand *why* something happens we're more strongly motivated to put our knowledge to good use.

Carcinogenic chemicals do their dirty work generally because they are molecules known as "free radicals," or because they produce free radicals in chemical reactions in the body. A free radical has unbound electrons, which can interact freely with nearby molecules, something like a live wire that may give off a small spark by itself but creates a gigantic arc if it finds a conductor. Such a conductor in the body is a cell membrane. When a free radical makes contact with it, the "jolt" changes the structure of the membrane and the energy may be passed on to the nucleic acids of the cell. Toxic by-products are produced and the cell may become cancerous.

We're exposed to free radicals every day. I've mentioned the dangers of chlorine: when it reacts with fluoride and other substances in our drinking water, free radicals result. The bromine in sea water, invading coastal lands as the water table falls, is known to produce free radicals in well water.

Free radicals also account for the suspected carcinogenic properties of polyunsaturated vegetable oils. Yes, these are the oils that have been recommended to us for the past 20 years by health authorities as a means of lowering cholesterol. I've discussed the pitfalls of the dietary cholesterol warning in the previous chapter. We now know that unsaturated fats are easily oxidized—that is, they lose a hydrogen ion, leaving behind the free negative charge that makes them free radicals. And this isn't mere chemical theory. Recent work by Drs. Morton Pearce and Seymour Dayton, a study of polyunsaturates for the control of atherosclerosis, turned up the ominous finding that subjects in the group fed margarines had double the cancer rate of the group fed butter.

Now we can see the importance of a vitamin like E. It's an antioxidant. In nature, vegetable oils are always accompanied by vitamin E: as rapidly as the oil oxidizes, giving up a hydrogen ion, E is there to donate a new one and thus prevent the molecule from becoming a free radical. The danger is that some polyunsaturate oils remain in the body for months, "time bombs" constantly threatening to generate free radicals. The good news is that if the vitamin E in your food sources isn't sufficient to counteract the oxidation of polyunsaturates, supplemental E can be taken. *This vitamin is also stored in the body.*

You will be hearing more about an obscure mineral, selenium, in the nutritional literature in the next few years because of its exciting antioxidant property in conjunction with vitamin E. A growing body of evidence indicates that this trace mineral, one of the most poisonous substances on earth but essential in small quantities in the body, could well be the most potent protection against both heart disease and cancer.

The rapidly mounting research on selenium is well worth summarizing. At the Cleveland Clinic Foundation, Drs. Charles E. Willis and Raymond J. Shamberger found in 1971 that where selenium was highest in the soil the surrounding area had the lowest incidence of heart disease and cancer. Selenium is distributed quite unevenly on the earth's surface, probably because it was deposited by ancient volcanoes and leached into now-dried-up basins. South Dakota has such a high level, for example, that some grazing animals are poisoned by it, while Ohio is very deficient and requires selenium supplements in cattle feed. Further studies by Drs. Shamberger and Douglas Frost showed that the residents of Rapid City, South Dakota, have the lowest cancer rate in the United States, while those in Lima, Ohio, have twice that rate. Shamberger and Willis analyzed blood levels of selenium and cancer deaths per 100,000 population in 19 cities and found that the selenium correlated almost in a linear progression with the cancer death rates: the lower the selenium, the higher the death rate.

Selenium has also shown surprising effectiveness in laboratory tests. In 1974 Dr. Gerhard Schrauzer found that the incidence of breast cancer in susceptible female mice was reduced from 82 percent to 10 percent merely by adding trace amounts of selenium to their drinking water. The tumors that did occur were delayed and were less malignant. Several studies have also been done of the effect of selenium against carcinogens added to the diet of laboratory animals. Dr. Richard Passwater determined that selenium and other antioxidants reduced stomach cancer in rats from 85 percent to 15 percent. Dr. John R. Harr and colleagues fed groups of 20 mice both carcinogens and varying amounts of selenium over a 210-day period. Those mice receiving little or no selenium had an 80 percent cancer rate; those receiving a relatively high amount of selenium had only a 10 percent rate; and the group receiving the highest selenium dosage had a bare 3 percent rate of cancer. Dr. Lee Wattenberg and Drs. C. G. Clayton and C. A. Baumann have reported similar findings in carcinogen experiments with laboratory animals.

Statistical comparisons of populations outside the United States also point to the effectiveness of selenium against cancer of many kinds. Venezuela has a high selenium concentration in its soil in comparison with the United States, as does Japan. Cancer of the large intestine occurs with a mortality of about 13 per 100,000 persons in the United States, but only 3 per 100,000 in Venezuela. Japan has an extremely low breast and lung cancer rate in comparison with the United States. Surely there are other dietary variables, but, in the absence of other differences between these countries as striking as that of selenium soil content, these are important clues.

Selenium, in fact, may turn out to be more important than vitamin E in cancer prevention. So far, it seems to be most effective in conjunction with E. A synergistic effect by the two was suggested in a study by Drs.

John Martin of Colorado State and Julian E. Spallholz of the Long Beach, California, Veterans Administration Hospital. Dietary selenium and vitamin E taken together significantly enhanced the primary and secondary production of antibodies: with a dosage of 0.7 parts per million selenium, antibodies were increased sevenfold; at 2.8 parts per million, antibodies went up thirtyfold. The next few years promise confirmation of all this work and the exploration of many other facets of this long-neglected trace mineral.

What should you do in the meantime? Dr. Schrauzer says, "The key to cancer prevention lies in insuring the adequate intake of selenium, as well as other essential trace elements." In view of the generally low levels of selenium in the soil of the United States, Dr. Passwater says it would be "suicidal" not to take a dietary selenium supplement. Some day, it may be necessary to get a reading on the soil content of your locale. I recommend that women especially, because of the possibility of breast cancer, take a vitamin/mineral supplement that contains selenium (about 50 micrograms). The proper level is important: a five- or tenfold increase in this dosage can cause damage to nerve cells. If you take a high-potency vitamin pill with chelated minerals, make certain it also contains selenium within a safe range.

Cancer Risk in the Diet: Too Much Smoke and No Fiber

Diet is a close companion of lifestyle, and the American lifestyle is largely characterized by a death wish manifested by use of cigarettes and by a total complacency over the fiber content of diet.

There is no magic pill—not vitamins C or E, not selenium—that can compensate for gross risks in your lifestyle. The two most important are smoking and lack of dietary fiber. A few well-chosen examples should convince you that popping a pill is no substitute for good sense.

If you're accustomed to thinking of the risk of smoking only in terms of lung cancer, consider two recent studies that link cigarettes with the whole range of cancers. For these studies, Mormon populations were selected because they are the only easily identified nonsmokers. They also have a moderate lifestyle—no alcoholic beverages or caffeine—but these toxic substances have never been linked clinically or in chemical studies with cancers: by themselves, they aren't carcinogens.

Begin with the fact that Utah has the least incidence of cancer of any state in the Union. Utah's population is 70 percent Mormon. In 1976

Dr. Joseph L. Lyon enlarged on this correlation by comparing large numbers of Utah Mormons with Utah non-Mormons. It was expected that the cancers known to be induced by smoking would be much rarer among the Mormons. Surprisingly, Mormons also had significantly lower rates of cancers of the breast, uterus, cervix, ovary, stomach, and nervous system.

As if to take into account any variables that might have been due to living conditions in Utah, Dr. James E. Enstrom studied similar groups in California. An epidemiologist at UCLA, Dr. Enstrom reported in *Science* in 1977 that Mormons in California were better off relative to non-Mormons in their state than their Utah counterparts—perhaps because other Californians smoke more than non-Mormon residents of Utah. Their overall death rate was one-half that of non-Mormon Californians. Their death rate from cancer was somewhat less than one-half. And in specific cancers their death rate was as low as one-third.

Cancer of the colon and rectum is the second most common cancer in the United States. Fiber in the diet results in an effective preventive and possible purgative of carcinogens in the intestines (see Chapter 11 for a discussion of the role of fiber in our diets). An 8-gram daily fiber intake is sufficient for this cleansing, anticarcinogenic benefit. The current American diet averages about 4 grams—half of what's needed.

I say "possible" purgative of carcinogens because the research in this field, as in many others in preventive medicine, is incomplete. It's all right for the American Cancer Society to state that 75 percent of the carcinomas of the colon and rectum could be prevented by early diagnosis and treatment; but *preventive medicine isn't merely early detection*. A carcinoma is a malignant tumor, especially one that tends to metastasize, or spread. One of every five people in the United States currently has polyps, or tumors, in the colon or rectum. Current research in preventive medicine is aimed at determining the cause of these cancers: there is growing suspicion that they are connected with high bacteria counts in stools and the activity of bile salts and fatty acids in conjunction with carcinogens in the diet. So it appears that colonic and rectal cancers can be controlled by keeping the natural elimination processes in the body in regular working order.

The key word here is "regular." The static accumulation of bacteria on the linings of the intestines, due to various degrees of constipation, can be prevented with a diet rich in whole grains, nuts, raw vegetables, and fresh fruit. As we will see in Chapter 11, it is the non-natural food diet that is responsible for irregularity in the bowels and all the diseases, including cancer of the colon and rectum, associated with such irregularity.

The Courage to Believe in Your Own Body

The message I've tried to present in this chapter is that the resources of your own body are your first and perhaps your best line of defense against cancer. Of course you must have confidence in your doctors. You must avail yourself of their advice and the whole array of therapies at their disposal. At the same time, be aware of the overreliance on technology in dealing with your problem. One of the most encouraging signs in the present transitional phase in medicine is a disenchantment with tools, techniques, and drugs in treating even such life-threatening diseases as cancer. In the recent past we have seen enormously expensive pieces of equipment brought to bear on diagnostic problems—to measure, examine, record, analyze. Such equipment is seductive to the physician, who wants to know. It's comforting to the patient (and the insurance pays for it anyway, we think). It's profitable to just about everybody. The trouble with gold-plated medical practice is not merely that the nation can't afford it but that it can easily blind us to the basic obligation we have to heal ourselves.

Have I convinced you that the nutritional approach to illness—even to cancer—comes first? Perhaps the weight of authority, of conventional medical practice, still deters you. An argument from authority is the weakest argument of all, but as a final incentive to embrace the nutrition prescription let me point out what some very knowledgeable people think about what I've discussed so far in this book:

Dr. Arthur Upton, director of the National Cancer Institute, states: "I take vitamin C and a multiple vitamin preparation; I do not drink heavily, although I'll have an occasional drink. I minimize my intake of animal fat. I also take a substantial amount of fiber, including a large amount of green leafy vegetables, and I eat bran for breakfast and try to control my weight. I guess you might say I try to hedge my bets."

Dr. Thomas J. Slaga, head of the Skin Carcinogenesis and Tumor Prevention Group at Oakridge National Laboratory, says: "I drink a lot of orange juice. I eat a lot of vegetables like cauliflower and things that have certain flavones that may have an inhibitory effect against cancer."

Dr. Ernst L. Wyndner, well-known cancer researcher and president of the American Cancer Foundation: "I think a high-fiber diet is important in preventing colon cancer."

Dr. Fred Rapp, chairman of the Pennsylvania State University College of Medicine and director of the Specialized Cancer Research Center, says he gave up smoking ten years ago. "In a department I chair with 75 people," he adds, "we no longer have an authentic smoker."

Dr. Linus Pauling: "I take 10 grams of vitamin C, 25,000 units of vitamin A, and good amounts—several times the MDRs—of other vitamins. I abstain from smoking and take some regular exercise. I believe, from the existing evidence, that practices of this sort can decrease the incidence of cancer by as much as 75 percent."

The example a patient recently gave me may add up in your mind as more persuasive than any of the above.

Everything about Leslie V. pointed to insurmountable odds in her battle against cancer. At the age of fifty-five she was found to have breast cancer. Her mother had died of cancer. Her emotional and financial states were in shambles as a result of preexisting disease of her gallbladder, a disturbed heart rhythm, and a divorce. Her physician urged immediate surgery of her left breast. Instead, Leslie armed herself with all the nutritional information she could get and embarked on a supplement program of proteolytic enzymes, vitamins, and substitution of other foods for meat. The cancer didn't go away—but neither did it spread. Three years later she had a simple excision of the tumor. Now, five years later, there is no sign of cancer.

When she came to me, five years after she should have been dead according to the statistics, I found her supplemental program quite good: 50,000 units of vitamin A, 5 to 10 grams of vitamin C, 1,200 I.U. of vitamin E, and a general vitamin and mineral pill. Her immediate problem of irregularity I found traceable to low magnesium. With a series of gradually increasing doses of this mineral she arrived at the right level to be able to do away with laxatives and enemas.

What struck me most about this case was Leslie's confidence in her own body's power to heal. Perhaps she was motivated to treat herself by religious beliefs that she held in the importance of inner strength. I know that she has found a sense of purpose now in bringing her nutritional knowledge to others who face cancer. I hope that through the medium of this book her courage will move many of you to find that there is plenty you can do about cancer.

The Nutrition Prescription for Cancer

- For prevention, make unprocessed foods a bigger part of your diet and be sure to include plenty of crude fiber
- Increase selenium food sources, such as whole grains and beans, as well as vitamin E, at least 400 units per day
- Take a complete micronutrient supplement and plenty of extra vitamin C
- Avoid excessive protein, epecially in aged beef and poultry, which are high in microorganisms associated with cancer
- Avoid excess dietary fat, particularly heated or cooked fats, which form carcinogens and free radicals
- When treatment is already indicated, be sure to explore nutritional approaches, even in conjunction with traditional therapy
- In particular, vitamins A and C in large doses and supplements of trace minerals may be helpful
- In general, avoid unnecessary exposure to notorious cancer-causing substances: smoking, radiation, some food additives, some industrial chemicals

7

The Sugar Disease: Hypoglycemia, Diabetes, and Dietary Suicide

When I was growing up, the only warning we got about sugar was that it would "rot your teeth." We now know that it's not sugar itself that rots teeth, but lactic acid, which the oral bacteria make from sucrose (the chemical name for table sugar). And sugar immobilizes a natural cleansing mechanism in the teeth and so allows lactic acid to destroy enamel. Healthy teeth can rot quickly with any breach in the enamel in such circumstances.

Our cravings for sugar are also deceptive. A "sweet tooth" is nothing less than an addiction, which has been fostered in the public at large by the inclusion of sugar in almost every processed supermarket item, for the food industry has discovered that high-sugar items are hugely successful in the marketplace. At the same time, sugar is one of the cheapest and most useful "fillers" in a processed food. These factors have combined to make sugar a staple instead of a seasoning, and, as we shall see, an insidious one.

There are two basic problems with table sugar that together lead to a host of problems, affecting the heart, the liver, the glands, and the bowels. First, it is devoid of any micronutrients and so promotes deficiencies when taken in large amounts. Second, the process whereby it becomes addictive is in itself damaging to various parts of the body. That process is called the hypoglycemic reaction.

Do we eat too much sugar? On the average, each of us takes in about one-quarter of our calories in the form of refined sugar. At 160 pounds per person, an American eats his weight in sugar each year.

The prominence of sugar in the human diet has only occurred in the last 150 years. The diet of primitive man was rich in micronutrients and did not include refined sugar of any kind. Because sugar's widespread use has only been recent, humans have not had time to develop a sugar tolerance. The fact is that most of us are sugar *in*tolerant and subject to an increased incidence of degenerative diseases in direct proportion to the amount of sugar we eat. Another difference between our diet and primitive diets (chiefly an agricultural diet) is that our ancestors consumed starch (about 400 grams of starch, close to a pound a day) while we eat *sugar* (about 150 grams per day). In the case of starch, the digestive process takes a fairly long time—two or three hours—whereas sugar takes under an hour, because it is a smaller molecule. Starch is made up of a long chain of glucose molecules, which are gradually released by digestive enzymes in the intestine, leading to a slow rise in blood glucose, a weak stimulus to insulin and other hormones. Sucrose is rapidly absorbed and causes a rapid rise in blood sugar, a strong stimulus to insulin and other hormones designed to keep blood glucose on an even keel. The other hormones thus stimulated—glucagon, adrenaline, and cortisone—also cause an unhealthy increase in fat and cholesterol in the blood, while overstimulation of insulin causes low blood sugar, also called hypoglycemia. The increase in triglyceride, a form of fat, thickens the blood and causes cells to clump, interfering with oxygen transport. In healthy people this makes for a sluggish feeling; in diseased coronary vessels it can precipitate heart attacks. The excess cholesterol tends to attach itself to weak or damaged areas of the blood vessel walls, thus initiating plaques that may eventually grow large enough to cut off flow through the vessel. (See Chapter 4 for a discussion of the full role of cholesterol in heart disease.)

Sucrose is a double sugar: one molecule of glucose and one of fructose. In nature, sucrose is found mostly in fruits, honey, sugar beets and sugar cane. Until the relatively recent farming of sugar cane and sugar beets, it had never been available in large amounts. An average daily intake of only 16 grams, the amount in a medium-sized fruit, was all one was likely to get. The fructose part of this came to an almost negligible 8 grams per day. As the average sucrose intake has risen to 150 grams per day, however, fructose has now increased up to 75 grams per day. Fructose, it appears, creates serious chemical problems in the human body. Dr. Linus Pauling comments, "There is little doubt that this great intake of fructose, to which human beings have been subjected only during the last century, is the cause of many of our ills."

Why? Because the larger amounts of fructose taken in sucrose have another action that leads to low blood sugar. Excessive amounts of fruit or fruit juices are, in this respect, as harmful as large amounts of table sugar. The fructose from sucrose blocks the release of glucose from glycogen (the substance the body stores for its future energy demands) in the liver. Without this source of glucose flowing into the bloodstream when needed the symptoms of low blood sugar appear, just as they do in the overproduction of insulin characteristic of hypoglycemia.

Fructose ingested *by itself,* however, is not known to cause hypoglycemia. In fact, it has been shown to be an effective substitute for sucrose for just this reason. Dr. Daniel Palm observed that when he exchanged 100 grams of fructose for sucrose, then blood cholesterol and blood fats were not elevated, and the amount of stress hormones decreased. This confirmed the welcome news that fructose caused less hormonal stress than did sucrose.

Since fructose is about twice as sweet as sucrose, less is required to satisfy our taste buds. For this reason it is likely that fructose will become more popular than sucrose before long—as it is in Europe now—possibly playing a valuable role in weight reduction.

Why Sugar Intake Causes Low Blood Sugar

Since sucrose is assimilated very quickly, the blood receives it very quickly. Normally, some very sensitive and delicate mechanisms, such as the action of insulin, keep your blood sugar level at a certain balance, and any increase in sugar or depletion of it triggers a balancing mechanism that restores this level to what is normal *for you.* Thus, when you eat sugar and your blood sugar level goes up, your pancreas secretes insulin to counteract the rise. The pancreas is the blood sugar level monitor, so to speak, and restores the balance. But this is the problem: the pancreas is a monumental overachiever, especially when it meets a sugar that is so quickly absorbed in the bloodstream. The insulin it shoots into your blood to counteract sugar overdose works so quickly that it creates a *drop* in blood sugar levels before a balance can be restored. This drop, in turn, results in a craving for more sugar: your body "tells you" your blood sugar is too low. The problem is that the body doesn't "know" this is only a temporary condition, and so you crave sweets. You take more sugar, which signals insulin release, again lowering the blood sugar level. In this cycle, the pancreas is overworked and worn out, which can lead to diabetes. Diabetes involves a constant high blood sugar level because you cannot get enough regulating insulin from your pancreas to lower it.

Long-term studies have been conducted with large groups of people who have changed their dietary sugar habits. From these we know that about one person in every six will eventually develop outright diabetes by adopting the present diet of Western civilization which is so high in sucrose and in refined carbohydrates. The number of people who are *pre-diabetic* and *pre-hypoglycemic* is more likely to be three out of five.

Dr. Aharon M. Cohen of Hadassah Medical Research Center in Jerusalem studied 6,000 immigrants from Yemen when they arrived in Israel in 1959, and followed them up 15 years later. There was negligible diabetes when they arrived, only three cases in 6,000 people. After 15 years on the Westernized sugar diet, about 1,000 cases of diabetes were found, one in every six people over age thirty. Two additional facts: the sugar intake in Israel is only half that in the United States, averaging 80 grams for the Yemenites in Israel compared to 150 grams here. The previous, traditional diet of the Yemenites was high in fat but low in sugar. This fact would also seem to dispose of dietary fat as a cause of diabetes. But sugar obviously is a cause of diabetes in what might be called susceptible individuals.

Dr. Cohen went a step further to demonstrate this relationship: he fed a Yemenite diet to laboratory rats and compared the results with another group on a Western-type diet. After just two months the blood sugar test showed some diabetes in those rats fed the high-sucrose, Western diet. Some animals remained relatively well, however, and others became seriously diabetic. Apparently there are greater individual differences in sugar tolerance than anyone even imagined.

Dr. Cohen then selectively bred a strain of rats from those that had the worst diabetes. After six generations, these diabetes-prone animals were divided again, some receiving a Yemenite diet and others a Western, high-sucrose diet. As was expected, those on the Western diet developed diabetes. Furthermore, Dr. Cohen found that these "susceptibles" became diabetic from a diet rich either in sucrose, glucose, or fructose. Diet and not heredity was clearly shown to be the key: "susceptible" rats from the same generation fed a Yemenite diet (starch but no sugar) remained free of diabetes. Dr. Cohen concluded that dietary sugar for humans should comprise no more than 5 percent of the total carbohydrate intake, or up to 3 teaspoons a day.

A critical finding of this study was that the level of sugar intake correlated directly with the onset of the disease. Dr. Cohen found that the rats became diabetic in only three weeks when on a diet with two-thirds of their calories as sugar. The rats stayed well for 13 weeks when sugar was only one-third of the calories. When the animals were placed on their normal diet again, the diabetes cleared up in a few days. When sugar feeding was resumed the diabetes occurred again, but this time it took only a few days instead of a few weeks.

These observations are borne out in my clinical practice. The first stage of overstimulation by dietary sugar leads to lowered levels of blood sugar, hypoglycemia. In susceptible individuals, continued stimulation leads to *permanently elevated* blood sugar levels, or diabetes. The situation in America is so bad that some authorities recommend that the glucose tolerance test be dispensed with as meaningless after age seventy because impaired sugar tolerance is so common. In other words, it is supposed to be normal to have high blood sugar, a diabetic condition, as part of growing old. This is one of those circular diagnoses by which anything common is considered normal and hence tolerable—like tooth decay.

How Do You Know When Sugar Is Getting the Better of You?

Within the last decade, after more than 50 years of the study of hypoglycemia around the world, the American Medical Association, the American Diabetes Association, and the Endocrine Society have issued separate statements to the effect that hypoglycemia is rare. More recently, some groups have claimed that the glucose tolerance test is of no diagnostic value. They have thus taken away the disease by taking away the only test that can accurately diagnose it. This test is valuable in almost any orthomolecular examination of a patient.

The methods doctors use to diagnose disturbances of blood sugar depend on their estimation of the seriousness of the "sugar disease." In most cases diagnosis is made by careful inquiry into the patient's symptoms and a thorough physical examination. Yet even at this level of concern diabetes is not obvious except in severe cases that are out of control, where the patient complains of excessive thirst and urination or emotional depression. Diagnosis is not easy because it is possible to attribute the symptoms to something else. I can't be sure of a diagnosis of diabetes without laboratory confirmation. A simple lab test for glucose in the urine is the most common clue, but only an abnormally high amount of glucose *in the blood* is conclusive.

It's possible for an early or mild case of diabetes to go undetected unless a complete study of the blood glucose levels is performed. A single blood sugar test done two hours after a meal will often suffice, since the blood sugar should return to normal at that point. But many physicians still prefer several blood samples taken at half-hour intervals for five hours after ingestion of a standard "meal" of 3.5 ounces of pure glucose. This is the glucose tolerance test; it is one of the important diagnostic tools in nutritional medicine.

The glucose tolerance test is invaluable not only in the diagnosis of diabetes and hypoglycemia, but also in less extreme cases to gauge the balance and integrity of the body chemistry. Since carbohydrate in the form of blood glucose is the normal fuel supply for the body's cells, it's obvious that proper delivery of this fuel is important to the function of every cell in the body. There is no other way at present to make a precise determination of blood glucose levels than by administering the glucose tolerance test. In the following chapter I will give some specific examples of how this test is used to analyze the broader effects of low blood sugar.

Again, keep in mind that sugar, like oxygen, is a basic fuel for all of the body's cells. This fact has been repeatedly misused by the sugar, candy, and cereal industries to promote their products. They conveniently ignore the hypoglycemic reaction, whereby *more* fuel ingestion can lead to *less* fuel in the bloodstream due to overstimulation of insulin. If something were to cut off your supply of oxygen without your knowing about it, how long would it take before you would feel panic? About 30 seconds! And you would be just as frightened to find yourself suffocating without a known cause as you would if you had choked on something or were under water too long. In fact, you might be more panicked if you didn't know the cause of your asphyxia.

Hypoglycemia is comparable to suffocation. As glucose is cut off or reduced, the body reacts with alarm. Since the entire reaction is chemical, hidden within the tissues of the body, few people are prepared to deal with their distressed emotions and cope with the culprit, low blood sugar. Most react by taking even more sugar, thus escalating the cycle.

If you're subject to frequent episodes of the symptoms of hypoglycemia, be prepared to eat a light nonsugar snack at an appropriate time.

Symptoms can be thought of here as *spells:* of hunger, dizziness, irritability, tremor, nausea, anxiety, and panic. Have your doctor administer a glucose tolerance test. Or, if the symptoms have already started, you can still reduce the extent of the stress by quickly drinking a glass of orange juice or eating a piece of fruit. If nothing else is available, even a teaspoon or two of sugar in a glass of water will help forestall symptoms. Sucrose is not a first choice, of course; but it will alleviate symptoms enough so that you can prepare a more wholesome meal to support your blood sugar level on a more even keel. Remember, your body makes all the sugar it needs from wholesome foods such as complex carbohydrates.

Micronutrients Can Help You Tolerate Sugar

Recent information confirms that micronutrients play an important role in sugar tolerance. First, it is known that hormones from the adrenal cortex, the glucocorticoids, are very sensitive to vitamin A deficiency. In mild or short-term cases, there will be a shortage of cortisone when vitamin A is in short supply because vitamin A is required for conversion of cholesterol into the adrenal hormones. And cortisone is the hormone that balances the effects of insulin.

Nutrition surveys have uncovered an alarmingly high incidence of vitamin A deficiency: one out of three school children in New York City, for instance. Other studies have shown that *vitamin A is quickly depleted by illness or stress,* due to the body's requirements for hormone and protein synthesis. Without doubt, most of us need vitamin A supplements in these circumstances in order to prevent permanent weakening of the adrenal glands and impairment of our ability to resist stress. Vitamin A also suppresses allergy, and it's quite possible to have an allergic reaction to sugar in ways other than hypoglycemia.

The micronutrients in the foods we eat instead of candy, soft drinks, and table sugar may, in fact, be more important than the mere avoidance of sucrose. This may help explain why natural starches, in potatoes and whole-grain cereals, are also known to be well tolerated by hypoglycemic patients.

Vitamin C is as important as A in the utilization of sugar. In 1977, Dr. Fred Dice of Stanford University reported that the dose of insulin required to control the sugar level in a juvenile diabetic who lacked the ability to produce insulin was cut in half by taking vitamin C in high doses.

Dr. Rex Clements, Director of the Clinical Research Center at the University of Alabama, found that diabetics lose more than normal amounts of inositol in their urine. The inositol has to compete with glucose for reabsorption in the kidney, and loses out. By employing a high-inositol diet, diabetics were able to maintain normal blood levels of inositol even though urinary output was increased tenfold. In the 15 cases he studied thoroughly, Dr. Clements found a statistically significant improvement in nerve function, an important measure in diabetes, on a high-myoinositol diet. This diet consists of increased intake of cantaloupe, peanuts, grapefruit, and whole grains.

Drs. Perla Miranda and David L. Horowitz found that a high-fiber diet lowered plasma glucose in insulin-dependent diabetics. Average sugar levels were 170 in the low-fiber intake group of 3 grams per day and 120 milligrams per 100 milliliters in the high-fiber diet group of 20 grams per day. The latter was crude fiber, such as in a high-fiber bread.

One reason why a high-fiber diet, consisting of crude fiber from grains and plants, might be effective in treating diabetes is that *fiber brings significant amounts of micronutrients, particularly chromium, into the diet.* There are good indications that chromium is essential to the utilization of glucose. The exact mechanism is not yet known, but the effect is so powerful that researchers Dr. Walter Mertz and later Dr. Henry Schroeder dubbed this "the glucose tolerance factor."

Dr. Schroeder's study of tissue levels of chromium indicates there is often chromium depletion in diabetics. Those who are dependent on a diet with high sugar and refined carbohydrates should be sure they are getting enough chromium. Not only does the American diet fall short of replenishing our chromium needs, but the presence of excessive amounts of sucrose probably increases our requirements by overstimulating the release of insulin.

My experience has been that hypoglycemia is extremely common in my patients. There are some patients who have a normal glucose tolerance test but marked clinical symptoms of hypoglycemia, particularly after eating high-carbohydrate foods. Tragically, many of these patients are children whose diets include "breakfast candy," cereals with more than 50 percent of their weight in sucrose and other sugars, as well as the junk foods that are dispensed in school cafeterias. When will we face the fact that the sugar business thrives on an addiction encouraged in the ignorant or defenseless?

The Nutrition Prescription for the Sugar Diseases

• Think of sugar as more than a bad habit—in reality, it is a cause of many diseases

• To help break a sugar craving, concentrate on specific micronutrients sugar is depriving you of: chromium, B vitamins, and magnesium in particular

• Counter the effects of sugar with more fiber to delay absorption

• Avoid excessive amounts of fruit and fruit juices

• When sweetening is necessary, use natural sugars, such as honey, for the micronutrients they also contain

• Remember, fructose is sweeter than sucrose, so you need less

8

Mental Disorders:
The Orthomolecular Alternative

When a doctor espouses a cause, a reader has a right to be skeptical. In a scientific field like medicine, issues are supposed to be decided by laboratory tests and clinical evidence. It would seem, therefore, that, when a small segment of the medical community is out of step with the vast majority of doctors, laypeople should be cautious about listening to special pleading. A single doctor or a small group of researchers can be self-deceived by their own promising but limited results. The placebo effect ("expecting helps make it so") exists for doctors as well as for patients.

I preface the discussion of mental illness with these remarks because this is a field in which measurement of results is perhaps the least scientific. Yet I've been in a fortunate position in the study of mental illness precisely because of this limitation: my entire career prior to specialization in orthomolecular medicine was involved in the use of placebos in psychotherapy and hypnosis. As I moved from traditional psychiatry to the nutritional factors in mental illness, I was already prepared by my experience with hypnosis and suggestibility to see the impact of psychic expectations of success. I hope to show in this chapter that, contrary to what a skeptic might feel about such an "unscientific" subject, the study of the nutritional basis of mental illness has yielded some of the most convincing results in the whole field of nutrition.

Breaking the Mind-Body Barrier

It seems logical enough to assume that mental troubles should be tackled by a mental activity: hence "talk therapy" for mental illness. So it was that when Drs. Abram Hoffer and Humphry Osmond began treating schizophrenia with niacin therapy they were greeted with derision by the psychiatric fraternity. Ironically, this was the beginning of *orthomolecular medicine,* and yet the resistance to change is still greater in psychiatry than in any other field discussed in this book.

Although various states and the federal government have authorized experimental programs of orthomolecular psychiatry, the faculties of universities and the staffs of leading institutions concerned with mental illness have traditionally ignored this alternative to conventional treatment. Consider what this sort of intransigence does to the bewildered relatives of patients.

Not long ago a colleague of mine began exploratory tests on a young man who was suffering from depression and possibly schizophrenia. He had been treated for a number of years as an outpatient at a hospital and was living in a halfway house for mentally disturbed young people. In desperation his parents had brought him to an orthomolecular psychiatrist: their son continued to threaten suicide and refused to converse with any doctor or nurse for any length of time. Finally, the Thorazine medication the young man was taking began to have serious side effects—an uncontrollable tightening of the facial muscles and impairment of vision. While the results of the glucose tolerance test and hair analysis were being awaited, the parents thought to mention this alternative they were exploring to the counselors at the halfway house. Immediately a conference was arranged with the psychiatrist in charge of the hospital's program, and the confused parents were informed that they would have to make a choice on the spot: drop the orthomolecular psychiatrist or take their son out of the hospital program! Feeling like heretics being banished from a church, they reluctantly decided to try the nutritional approach. It turned out their son was in fact suffering from severe mineral deficiencies and hypoglycemia and responded well to dietary treatment. Consider: if experienced psychiatrists and psychologists and nutritionists can't bridge the chasm between their various fields of interest, how are laypeople supposed to choose between them, especially when given an ultimatum?

Not all mental illness is nutritionally caused, of course; but it shouldn't be surprising that *much of it is*. Severe nutritional deprivation can leave permanent aftereffects in the nervous and hormonal systems. We can detect these defects through the glucose tolerance test, because it is a good indicator of metabolic adaptability. Exactly how biochemical changes affect the brain is an exciting new field but I will limit myself to the results I have seen in my own practice.

I turned to orthomolecular practice only after observing gross deficiencies in vitamins and minerals in many of my psychiatric patients and rapid improvement in those patients as a result of nutritional therapy. Then I had to ask myself: how much a factor in these cases was my own suggestibility? I have had quite a bit of experience in behavioristically oriented hypnotherapy. The placebo effect there is far greater than in nutrient therapy, so I was prepared for my patients' suggestibility and I could discount it accordingly. The question that kept coming back was this: How effective are *various* psychiatric approaches *independent of my personality?* I always question my objectivity in evaluating the success of my work.

I decided to resolve the question by asking 200 of my patients what they thought about the total treatment under my care. Since this study was accomplished by means of a rather lengthy questionnaire, it was to be expected that only 100 responded. I went over the age, sex, outcome, and diagnosis of those who did reply as compared to those who did not and was pleased to find that the two groups were comparable. I satisfied myself that the responders were not simply my best patients; in other words, the sample of patients was valid.

The patients were asked to indicate whether they felt any or all of the following treatments, all of which are employed in my practice, were beneficial:

1. A complete program of orthomolecular nutrition
2. Megavitamins
3. Orthocarbohydrate diet
4. Psychotherapy
5. Hypnosis
6. Drug therapy

I simplified the number of diagnostic categories to merely three: anxiety, depression and schizophrenia. Which illnesses responded to which therapies?

Far more patients rated orthomolecular or nutrition therapy as more valuable than any other form of therapy. The other therapies showed wide ranges of helpfulness, depending on the illness. Megavitamin therapy was rated valuable by only a small number of patients whose primary symptoms were anxiety or depression, but by three-quarters of the patients whose symptoms were of a schizophrenic type. Optimal carbohydrate regulation (which will be described fully in Chapter 15) was rated valuable by only a small number of my schizophrenic-type patients, while about half of those with anxiety and depression found it to be beneficial. One surprise for me in this follow-up was the high percentage who found that psychotherapy, just talking with their doctor and maintaining a good relationship with him as a concerned friend, was important in their recovery. In fact, psychotherapy was about as effective as the nutritional approach for schizophrenia and was rated considerably higher than hypnosis, including direct suggestion and relaxation training. Drug therapy was rated beneficial by about half as many patients as those who valued psychotherapy. The "art" of medicine is here to stay.

The results of this questionnaire are similar to those of a follow-up study of the parents of autistic children—that is, children with severe impairment of their language and personality development. Bernard Rimland, a psychologist who has pioneered in orthomolecular research and treatment for the past 15 years, reported that high-dosage vitamin therapy was rated as a positive benefit by these parents in two-thirds of his cases. Only one of four parents rated drug therapy as beneficial. Furthermore, almost a third of the children on drug therapy were felt by their parents to have been made worse by the medication. Megavitamins were associated with worsening of symptoms in only 3 percent of the cases.

There is an unfortunate tendency to take an either/or approach to the treatment of mental disorders. In reality, all therapies offer some help and there is no need to take sides as if this were a political issue. Nutritional and orthomolecular factors are important in *every case* of mental disorders, *every day*. They are the foundation for the basic health and well-being that make psychotherapy of any constructive kind possible. Equally important, in any serious mental illness *some* form of psychotherapy is necessary for complete treatment.

When to Choose an Alternative

If alternatives to drug therapy and reliance on psychotherapy are successful for many people, the only critical question about choice is safety. It is well established that vitamin therapy, even at high doses, is remarkably safe. While there have been a few cases of bad effects from prolonged exposure to high doses of vitamins A and D, these are not used in megavitamin therapy. Any bad effects of the B vitamins and ascorbate are quickly recognized and harmless: nausea, diarrhea, skin rash, or headache. These symptoms discourage further intake of the vitamins at high dosage and they clear up when dosage is reduced. In a number of cases megadoses of niacin have been observed to raise blood sugar and uric acid levels and, on rare occasion, to irritate the liver.

Megavitamins—or megadoses of micronutrients—do work. They work especially well in serious mental illnesses, such as the schizophrenias in adults and the autism-type disorders of children. Anxiety and depression also will respond in some cases. While the B vitamins, particularly niacin and pyridoxine, are most beneficial, other B vitamins and vitamin C are also known to provide significant health benefits in large doses. And, while it is known that megavitamin therapy is one of the safest therapies we know of in psychiatric circles, it is unwise to undertake such treatment without your doctor's prescription and observation. It is important to know whether you are one of those unlucky few who are unable to tolerate large doses of vitamins and minerals comfortably or safely.

With the reservation of safety, then, there is no reason why one shouldn't explore every possible avenue of psychiatric relief. Unfortunately, as the following examples will show, in the past most patients have come to orthomolecular therapy only as a last resort.

Fear of Father or Addiction to Sugar?

Alex was a twenty-five-year-old man who had been disabled by chronic anxiety and depression for the previous five years when he consulted me. He had always been outgoing, fearless and a leader among his peers. He had been a champion wrestler at nineteen and spent his summers working at heavy labor. Accustomed to pushing himself, he planned an unusual vacation hitchhiking 1,000 miles without a break. He kept awake by taking caffeine pills and drinking cola beverages.

After a day and a half, only halfway to his destination, he suddenly had his first anxiety attack. He found himself nervous and uncomfortable around people. He was shaken by this change in mood and worried that he was becoming paranoid. He somehow managed to get back to his home in San Francisco, where he stayed under his parents' care for some time. His symptoms continued to worsen and he consulted the first of his three psychiatrists, a traditional orthodox Freudian analyst, who saw him regularly for the next three years.

During this time Alex had no relief from his symptoms except by taking strong tranquilizers. Then he put himself on a vegetarian diet. Within a few weeks he improved enough to get out of the house, get a job, and visit his old girlfriend. On one occasion, however, his car broke down a few hundred miles from home and his symptoms returned. Housebound again, he returned to analytic therapy for another year even though he felt it was not helpful. His analyst told him his symptoms were due to "fear of your father."

Then one day he read about vitamin therapy and decided to try it. After he took B-complex vitamins, there was an almost immediate improvement. Then his analyst told him he would get sick from the vitamins, so he stopped taking them. As soon as he stopped the vitamins, he got worse again. That did it. He quit therapy and consulted another doctor, this time a Jungian analyst. Within two months his anxiety was much worse. This time he had a full-blown anxiety attack with difficulty in breathing. His new analyst interpreted this as due to "breaking off the negative transference" with his old analyst. In desperation Alex again started taking his B-complex vitamins. Again he experienced relief. This convinced him to seek orthomolecular therapy, and he came to see me.

Dietary analysis now replaced psychoanalysis. My interpretation: too much sugar. Though not obese, he ate more than two-thirds of a pound of sucrose a day and almost a pound of carbohydrate. Upon giving up sugar, he experienced immediate improvement, sufficient enough to allow him to discontinue the tranquilizer he had been taking every day for the past five years! The dietary analysis also revealed that at the beginning of his illness his diet had been even worse. At that time he was working 70 hours a week and taking 3 hours of classes a night. He often went without sleep and drank a dozen or more cups of coffee a day, each with a heaping teaspoonful of sugar. That's about 80 grams of sucrose just in the coffee. He usually skipped breakfast and ate only a sandwich on white bread for lunch. Dinner was ample, but inadequate for his needs. Finally, just before the anxiety attack that heralded his illness, he took 12 caffeine tablets while eating only vending machine foods, soft drinks, and coffee.

I ordered a glucose tolerance test even though his blood and urine sugars had always been within normal limits. The results were startling: he was fully diabetic. The sum of blood glucose values while fasting at a half hour, one hour, and two hours was 934 milligrams per 100 milliliters. A score of 800 indicates clinical diabetes. There was no danger of coma, but at the third hour his sugar level plunged dangerously low and was accompanied by a relapse of his symptoms, weakness, dizziness, and tremor. He felt depressed for a full day after the test. Clearly, his symptoms were caused by blood sugar changes. He *learned more about his illness in five hours of the glucose tolerance test than he had in five years of psychoanalysis.*

Treatment included a complete regimen of vitamins and mineral supplements. There was no additional improvement, as he had resumed vitamins on his own before consulting me. After two weeks of evaluating micronutrient factors, I introduced him to my orthocarbohydrate (OC) diet. This diet demonstrates the physical and emotional effects of varying carbohydrate intakes from zero to a few hundred grams per day. The trick is to stay at an almost zero-carbohydrate intake long enough to persuade the body to burn fat. One of the products of fat burning is acetone, which, with its two companion molecules, is known as ketone. The ketones appear in the blood and urine of anyone when fasting or avoiding carbohydrate foods; when the ketones are present in measurable quantities, this chemical condition is known as "ketosis."

Alex felt so well in ketosis, at a low carbohydrate intake, that he went against my orders and stayed on low carbohydrates longer than the initial five-day limit I normally prescribe. Fortunately, he experienced no adverse reaction. (The reason for this limit is that a few people are susceptible to irregular pulse if they deplete their minerals, particularly potassium and sodium. If this should happen it is easily corrected by taking a potassium supplement or perhaps drinking some orange juice, which provides potassium and enough carbohydrates to terminate the ketosis state.)

After two weeks in ketosis, Alex felt truly well for the first time in years. The anxiety spells that had formerly occurred several times a day were almost entirely absent. In the next few months he experienced further improvement by the use of calcium supplements, which he found useful in reducing the few anxiety spells he still had. (Some authorities feel that calcium supplements combat anxiety by inactivating lactic acid, a by-product of glucose in the body chemistry.) Further, he found that the B vitamin niacinamide was noticeably helpful in stabilizing his mood and restoring his confidence. He maintained his diet at only 60 grams of carbohydrates during this time and lost 30 pounds before his weight finally stabilized at 150 pounds, optimal for his height of 5 feet 10 inches.

Within six months he had moved out of his parents' home and found a new girlfriend. Needless to say, his mood improved along with his self-confidence. Although he still had a way to go to regain his former level of ease and complete freedom from anxiety, there was no doubt he would make it. I gave him some instruction in self-hypnosis, which helped him make the move to his new apartment, but then referred him for behavioristic psychotherapy to support the coming months of rehabilitation. The outcome was so successful that his behavior therapist published a report of the case in a professional journal a year later. His conclusion was that counter-conditioning had proved successful where five years of previous attempts at therapy had failed. Nutrition took a back seat in this naïve behavioristic interpretation.

Alex's comments on my follow-up questionnaire include the following: "I don't believe that I could have recovered without correcting the metabolic and nutritional disorder. Also, there is no doubt in my mind that orthomolecular therapy and your diagnosis [of diabetes] saved my life. Without it I could never have recovered and would probably either have committed suicide or been institutionalized to mull over my childhood for the rest of my life."

I think it's reasonable to suggest that anyone who has persistent symptoms of anxiety, depression, fatigue, headache, impairment of concentration or memory, allergy, or any psychosomatic condition should have a glucose tolerance test as part of his medical evaluation. In particular, I wish that psychiatrists and counselors dealing with sexual problems would think of this with anyone who is impotent. I'll never forget the unnecessary suffering I shared with one particularly likable young husband who, along with his devoted and lovely wife, couldn't understand their total lack of sexual relations. This was 15 years ago, before I was treating with mega-nutrition and before Linus Pauling had coined the word "orthomolecular." I dare say if my former patient were treated today, even after all this time, there is a chance that mega-nutrition might restore his potency. At least this knowledge might have spared him some of the expense and stress of soul-searching for the hidden conflict or subconscious fear or anger that stood in the way of happiness and fulfillment—and which we were helpless to remedy at the time. Today we know that impairment of the function of the glands and of the brain is quite possible in persistent hypoglycemia.

The importance of a glucose tolerance test was underscored in my early experience in the case of twenty-year-old Evelyn W., daughter of a mathematics professor. A slow learner as a child, she had experienced mental dullness and depression for many years. She still had difficulty distinguishing left from right. Nevertheless, she managed to complete two years of college before finding that the pressures of study were overwhelming. She was unable to muster enough energy to hold even a menial job for more than a few months. Then her symptoms got worse: she had put herself on a vegetarian diet and it lacked enough eggs and dairy products to assure adequate essential amino acids from protein. With vitamin and mineral supplements and adjustment of her carbohydrate intake she began to improve. Her optimal level was 90 to 120 grams of carbohydrate per day. She felt worse after a trial on the B vitamin, niacin. It caused her lips to crack and it took two weeks to clear them up.

The most remarkable finding in her case came from the glucose tolerance test. Her fasting blood sugar was normal and, after she ingested the glucose, her blood sugar rose only a bit higher than normal. It then came down a bit precipitously, but still within normal limits up to the second hour. At that time, a most unusual thing occurred: her blood sugar dropped almost to zero at two and a half hours and was undetectable at three hours. At only three and a half hours, she recovered. Her self-description of this event: "The test wasn't as bad as I expected." She forgot to take her notes during this time, which I had asked her to do, and more detailed questioning revealed that she had gone into a trance—she had completely blanked out. I suspect this sort of experience was so common in her life that she did not regard it as foreign. However, had the hypoglycemia been more prolonged, she might have gone into a coma or had an epileptic seizure. Luckily, her brain wave test revealed no tendency to epilepsy. This case shows that even severe hypoglycemia can be missed unless a glucose tolerance test is performed. Evelyn responded well to a typical low-sugar, low-carbohydrate diet.

The drowsy mental state and lethargy of the pre-diabetic is often overlooked as due to some other cause. In fact, it is usually the result of an excessive amount of insulin generated by abnormally high blood sugar. Of the supposedly normal population of the country who think of themselves as healthy and disease-free, only half have a normal response to the glucose tolerance test. The rest may not be diabetic or hypoglycemic, but they exhibit an irregular pattern indicative of many other potential problems. In the first hour their blood sugar may go unusually high, a pre-diabetic response; or it may drop too rapidly or too low in the three following hours. This response may indicate hypoglycemia or other problems that may add up to a serious condition taken together with other symptoms.

Insulin is used in the body to transport glucose to brain cells, and this fact explains a lot. It also affects one of the amino acids, tryptophane, which is quickly converted in the brain into a natural tranquilizer, serotonin. This makes you sleepy. Naturally this is a pleasant feeling if it happens at bedtime, but embarrassing if it happens at a party and dangerous if you are driving.

It is not uncommon for my patients to report that they cannot keep awake during the test. They usually lie down and go to sleep at the laboratory when their blood sugar reaches its low point, barely rousing themselves for the succeeding blood samples. These patients often have serious disturbances in their blood sugar regulation but are out of touch with it and rarely associate it with food. The majority of hypoglycemia sufferers have lost contact with the normal instinct in response to low blood sugar: hunger. Some patients experience severe mood changes during the low blood sugar response: weeping without any conscious reason can be most distressing and embarrassing. Anxiety and foreboding, irritability, anger, and outright paranoia have all occurred during these blood sugar episodes and often have helped my patients understand their symptoms for the first time.

In a hundred of my patients, selected at random, there was a *90 percent rate of blood sugar abnormality*. All of those with anxiety as a chief symptom had abnormal blood sugar, not always low, but most commonly with extra fluctuations mid-test. Each rise in sugar during the test comes from a surge of adrenaline and this causes the heightened anxiety response. Depressed patients were also likely to have an abnormal tolerance test. However, the depressed patients commonly had a flat curve or a drop in sugar to hypoglycemic levels. The flat curve indicates that the blood sugar level does not rise after drinking the sugar solution; the sugar is not promptly absorbed or the insulin is overly active, driving the ingested sugar out of the bloodstream too quickly. This type of response is known to occur in cases of hormonal disorders, such as weak or damaged adrenal glands and low thyroid conditions.

While I find no single type of glucose tolerance pattern in schizophrenia, I well remember a schizophrenic youth who consulted me several years ago. He had a flat curve with a late drop to reactive hypoglycemia. His sugar level was in the 80s for three hours and then dropped into the 40s. At this time he became quite irritable. In the hospital, where I evaluated his condition, I saw that nursing notes described him as generally cooperative and likable despite his aloofness. However, at times he seemed extremely irritable for no reason. He couldn't account for it himself; yet the least annoyance made him want to strike out at people. Since he was 6 feet 7 inches tall and weighed 250 pounds, this was quite frightening to all concerned. I observed that he had no established interests and passed the time by drinking tea, about 20 cups or more a day. Each cup had three or more teaspoons of sugar, since the sugar bin was available without restrictions to the patients.

Once again I found that a hospital staff wasn't prepared to accept this diagnosis; my orders to substitute health drinks with brewer's yeast and to restrict sugar seemed just another fad. The patient had been told by his psychiatrist that vitamins were quackery and of no value, so it was impossible to gain his full cooperation with orthomolecular therapy in the short time before he had to be transferred to a state hospital. It was heartbreaking for his parents, who had tried so hard to give him a chance at orthomolecular treatment even before this therapy was very well known. But this patient was just not ready to accept vitamin pills, since no one else on the ward took them and his psychiatrist had spoken against them. The pity of it was that his tissue levels of micronutrients must have been severely depleted. Blood tests showed abnormally low levels of the B vitamin folic acid. In spite of what I knew, I was helpless to intervene.

When All Else Fails, Call the Psychiatrist

What we are seeing in these examples (and thousands of others of which these are only representative) is that patients are being taken away from psychiatrists as the patients' problems are found to be nonpsychogenic—that is, caused by something other than the mind or the psyche. This is as it should be, and no traditional psychiatrist would see this fact as denigrating to his profession. When we knew little about other causes of mental illness, we had no recourse but to treat all anxieties, all depressions, all schizophrenias alike.

The point is this: someone is diagnosed as having an emotional problem when no other diagnosis can be made. When all other disorders are ruled out what is left is mental illness. It is therefore incumbent upon the practicing psychiatrist to be open to the possibility that his diagnosis is always subject to error. He should be willing to look for more definitive clues against this background. His measure should be, "Is there a known cause of the symptoms I observe?" As Carl Pfeiffer writes, in his massive study *Mental and Elemental Nutrients,* "This positive yardstick is applied constantly by the inquiring scientist and should be used more often in medicine. At present there probably isn't a Freudian psychiatrist (or psychologist) who could give a valid and scientifically acceptable answer to this simple question."

It's no wonder that Abram Hoffer says of Pfeiffer's contribution, "This book represents the wave of the future. . . . Standard psychiatry (tranquilizers and talk) has proven itself bankrupt."

My own experience with my patients, as reflected in the survey I have mentioned above, would force me to qualify that judgment. In espousing the cause of orthomolecular psychiatry, I can't ignore nearly 100 years of Freudian history, nor my own eyes and ears. Positive, practical, constructive psychotherapy can be of real value in every illness of man! On the other hand, even within the nutritional movement, if I may call it that, there is much that a reasonable man can disagree with or reserve judgment on. The subject of hyperactivity in children is a case in point.

The hyperactive child might well be thought of as a symbol of our society and of how our society deals with problems. We are prone to create names and illnesses to categorize and thus do away with essentially nonmedical problems. The first impulse is always to treat disturbing behavior with drugs, especially if persuasion is hopeless. After some years of unsuccessful treatment of this broad class of "mental illness" with drugs and talk therapy, along came Dr. Ben Feingold with a nutritional suggestion. Could it be that a whole generation of children had been exposed to something in their diet that was absent in previous generations? Dr. Feingold focused on the additives used to give color or to preserve food.

Dr. Feingold's success in treatment, especially with a low-salicylate diet, is noteworthy. Salicylates influence the nervous system, and aspirin is the most prominent salicylate. Yet I would question whether the removal of fruits from the diet is effective because it removes a source of salicylates or because it removes a source of simple sugar. In fact, I see a direct parallel between the controlling of carbohydrates in epilepsy and the success of the same technique in hyperactive behavior.

Dr. Sam Livingston was the first to suggest and use a ketogenic diet, one that employed ketosis to establish a proper carbohydrate intake, in the control of epilepsy. He noticed that even when seizures weren't fully controlled by this diet there was a noticeable improvement in the behavior of epileptic children. In severe cases of children with abnormal brain waves, the ketosis technique has proved to be invaluable. I would conclude from all this that once a nutritional diagnosis is made the matter isn't ended: food allergies and irritation from preservatives and colorants may be important, but excessive carbohydrates may be even more so.

Judy was seven years old when her adoptive parents noticed her falling behind in her third-grade class. She seemed to be well liked, but couldn't cope for more than 20 minutes: she was constantly talking and couldn't sit still. Easily confused in games, she fell behind her peers in physical activities of all kinds. She could skate on one roller skate but not two. Her teachers thought her intelligent because of her facility with words, but projects never got done and her attention span was brief. In group dancing a teacher noticed that Judy was unable to follow the lead. She began to throw tantrums.

Because she obviously had difficulty doing things in sequence, counselors advised an evaluation for a neurological disorder. The report: normal. Psychological tests confirmed the same thing; the report indicated only a deficiency in mathematical facility. An evaluation team concluded: ". . . We recommend psychotherapy for this girl to allow her to talk about her feelings of early maternal deprivation and abuse."

Within three months, Judy was brought to me for help. As I've said plainly at the start of this chapter, I have no reason to demean psychotherapy—it has been effective with perhaps 80 percent of my patients. And here was a case in which there was indeed much to talk about. Judy's natural mother had been a severe alcoholic, as were the mother's ten brothers and sisters. Most of the members of her tragic family had died of alcoholism or suicide.

A quick evaluation pointed to some severe nutritional problems, however, which overrode anything of a psychogenic nature. Judy craved carbohydrates and had an incessant thirst. Her father and mother were horrified to observe Judy vomit and return to eating as if she had an insatiable hunger. The Feingold diet had failed to change any of this.

I calculated her carbohydrate intake at almost 300 grams a day, surely an excessive amount. Of this 50 grams were in the form of table sugar! Almost another 100 grams consisted of refined carbohydrate, equivalent to about 25 teaspoonsful of sugar. Judy managed to shovel all this into her small body away from home, in the form of candy bars and soft drinks and white bread at the corner store or school cafeteria. Her mother was careful to maintain a decent diet at home, including vitamin supplements. A good point to remember: supplemental vitamins were hardly enough protection against this nutritional travesty. Hair analysis suggested some mineral deficiencies: manganese and chromium. But I knew instinctively that nothing would improve until the carbohydrates were brought into balance. Judy began a ketosis program, as described in Chapter 15.

One day without carbohydrates produced "magnificent" results, as her mother described it. Judy was immediately calmer and then a bit lethargic. After another day or so she reached the ketosis state, indicating that fat was being converted into other forms in her body. As she added milk and bread to the diet, at the 50-grams-a-day level, ketosis ended and she was quite well indeed. Finally, as soon as she reached 160 grams of carbohydrate a day the symptoms came back in full force; she was restless and irritable, overly talkative, unable to concentrate. We moved back to a lower level of carbohydrates.

Food additives, which had once caused flareups, now no longer bothered her. He physical coordination was greatly improved. She could roller-skate and also ride a two-wheel bike. Previously friendless, she was suddenly sought after; she was even out playing baseball with the boys. She boasted to her mother about the youngsters who used to push her around: "Now I push them around." Her mother was especially impressed with her stamina: "She doesn't cry, even when they throw dirt in her face."

An examination a year later showed that the ketosis diet was hardly just a happy accident. At 129 grams a day of carbohydrates, she could function perfectly: that was her "ortho" level. Her dietary fats were up to 57 percent of her caloric intake from 39 percent a year before; yet her blood cholesterol had risen negligibly from 160 to 167. Meanwhile, the critical blood fat, triglyceride, was at a record low of only 19 milligrams per 100 milliliters.

The Carbohydrate Factor in Mental Illness

A few startling cases like Judy's convinced me that excessive carbohydrates were far more important in mental disorders than anyone had previously realized. Notice that by "excessive" I mean *excessive for a particular individual;* individual differences are as critical here as they are in heart disease. Beyond a large quantity of carbohydrate, such as the 300 grams Judy had been taking a day, almost everyone could be expected to be affected. A few unlucky individuals are unable to tolerate less than even half that amount. Why? Because our hormone systems are so sensitive and vary so much from one person to the next. I believe that when the blood glucose level drops too quickly or too far it's the result of even slight variations in carbohydrate intake; and when that happens, of course, stress hormones are unnecessarily released. At present I don't see any other explanation for the success of the orthocarbohydrate diet.

An individual case can be quite impressive when it involves a careful exploration of all reasonable therapies. This is why the example of Karen R. was important to me in thinking through the orthocarbohydrate theory. This fifty-seven-year-old woman was happily married to an insightful psychotherapist. She had lived a life of constant battling against fatigue and depression, and her medical history pointed to obvious causes. Her mother had had tuberculosis during her pregnancy and Karen was born with a tubercular infection that failed to heal until adolescence. In her twenties she had serious bouts of asthma and allergic dermatitis, which were held in check with hormone treatments. Her skin, however, gradually became a patchwork of depigmentation. As she entered her forties, she was caught up in the new awareness of the importance of iron in women her age, but her multivitamin supplement was apparently insufficient and she turned to stimulants, amphetamines and barbiturates. She was still on these daily pills, after 17 years, when she was referred to me.

After several years of exploring every conceivable psychological explanation for her lethargy and depression, she and her husband had decided on nutritional therapy. It seemed to me at our first meeting that her frail condition was highly indicative of nutritional deficiency, but a physical examination turned up no clues except her unusually brittle fingernails. We reviewed her extensive attempts at psychotherapy. While we awaited the results of her glucose tolerance test, she showed some improvement by taking the strong ration of vitamin and mineral supplements that I prescribed.

Surprisingly, she did not turn out to have what is normally thought of as low blood sugar. Rather, her sugar curve was wildly unstable. After three hours a strong adrenaline reaction raised her blood sugar 50 points, higher than after the immediate ingestion of the glucose solution to start the test. As I have learned from this case and many others, an unstable glucose reaction responds best to the OC diet. At 60 grams of carbohydrate a day, the transition point for her from ketosis, she improved dramatically in vigor and mood. But when she reached 110 grams, she again became listless and depressed. By limiting her intake to a figure between those levels, she was literally cured—a word any doctor hesitates to use. She hasn't had the need to take a stimulant since that time.

I caution the reader, again, about leaping to the conclusion that all psychotherapy is passé and that mental illness is only a manifestation of physical deficiencies. Even when the OC diet works, it's often only one factor in a patient's recovery—unlike the above case. Yet, in my experience, I've consistently found that the OC diet is a *factor* in eight out of ten cases of mental disorders that I have treated.

In 1975 I summarized the experience I had with 73 patients suffering from anxiety, depression, or schizophrenia, in an article in the *Journal of Orthomolecular Psychiatry*. At that time, only two out of three patients of all types reported "they felt their best" when their carbohydrate intake was adjusted to the OC level. I should also point out that in the later survey I conducted of 100 patients with the extensive questionnaire mentioned at the beginning of this chapter, the OC diet was rated as effective by only 40 to 50 percent of those suffering from anxiety and depression and much lower by schizophrenics. Nevertheless, by any standard, these results are exceptional in the field of mental illness. While the OC diet failed to ameliorate the delusions and confusion of schizophrenia, I know that it reduced attendant anxiety and improved general mood in these patients. In short, this orthomolecular approach to mental illness is a not a panacea, or the only solution, but it certainly is an alternative no therapist should ignore.

In Chapter 15, I will present the OC diet as a general nutritional program, not for any specific illness. For the moment I should assure you that it is quite natural and safe. The experience of ketosis, of starting to burn your stores of fat, is a normal response to fasting for as little as a day or two. Some very lean individuals find a low carbohydrate intake to be stressful and quite uncomfortable; most overweight people experience just the opposite. The general rule I've discovered is that an intake of from 60 to 90 grams of carbohydrate a day is optimal for the majority of people. Those who jog or are otherwise physically active every day can easily take from 30 to 90 additional grams. A marathon runner I know thrives on what we normally think of as junk food: milkshakes, fast-food hamburgers, french fries two or three times a day; on the other hand, he runs well over 100 miles a week and eats lots of fresh fruits, vegetables, beans, and whole grains. This is one more reason for being physically active. But I believe the prudent approach is to get your eating habits into line first, rather than try to correct them with exercise. For the vast majority of us, including anyone concerned with such a basic mental disorder as moodiness, nutrition is the truest therapist we will ever have.

The Nutrition Prescription for Mental Disorders

- For depression, concentrate on improving micronutrients
- For anxiety, reduce carbohydrate intake, especially with the OC diet
- If you have done the preceding and still don't feel well, then look for causes of disorders in food allergies and pollutants
- Realize your nutritional program is enhanced by appropriate forms of "talk therapy," mood conditioning, biofeedback, Transcendental Meditation, or whatever fits in with your point of view

9

Depression, Depletion, and Pollution

Most people, whether healthy or not, have suffered at one time or another from depression, depletion, and pollution. I am lumping these problems together not only because they are so common and cause so much suffering but because, unfortunately, they are likely to be overlooked or misdiagnosed by health professionals. I have seen or heard about too many cases in which patients have either been considered hypochondriacal or else have had to find the cause of their malaise themselves. Because the "new medicine" is so attuned to nutritional and environmental factors it is likely that health professionals will begin to recognize the effects of depletion and pollution more and more.

Ten years ago I was inclined, like my colleagues in psychiatry, to believe that all cases of depression were due to underlying emotional conflicts. But with my introduction to nutritional medicine I began to realize that depression is actually one of the early signs of nutritional depletion. Dr. Robert Kinsman and Dr. James Hood documented this in their classic study of vitamin C deprivation in human subjects. They found that mood depression was present in every case of vitamin C deprivation when the level of stored vitamin C was reduced by a third. A vitamin C-deficient diet produced this condition in only two to six weeks!

When I studied deficiency disease in more detail I came to realize that almost all nutrient and caloric deficiencies produced depression long before they produced physical illness. Lacking obvious physical signs, it is almost impossible for a physician to make a correct diagnosis —unless he happens to be an orthomolecular physician and takes a careful dietary history.

Postpartum Depression and "Female Problems"

Perhaps the most glaring example of depletion and the failure of traditional medicine to recognize it as such is the range of disorders we euphemistically call "female problems." That so diverse a group of illnesses—including menstrual disorders, menopausal problems, various infections, growths and pains and their associated anxieties and dysperceptions—are grouped under one label most surely reveals how little we must really know about these problems.

The role of nutrient depletion in these conditions has also been grossly oversimplified. For example, iron deficiency has been widely publicized by drug companies as a common problem among menstruating women. But iron supplementation for "tired blood" has served to distract women and their doctors from other equally prevalent and serious nutrient shortages.

The hormonal tides drain a woman's body of substantial amounts of blood cells and uterine cellular matter that must be regenerated. This regeneration uses up vitamins, such as folic acid, B_{12}, and B_6, as well as zinc, protein, and iron. The most common deficiency I have seen in women is that of folic acid. In addition, more women than men seem to go through a cycle of crash dieting for weight loss; this further aggravates their nutritional depletion.

These nutrient losses first result in fatigue, loss of mental concentration, and mood depression and not, as generally suspected, anemia. Other symptoms, such as water retention, commonly associated with the premenstrual syndrome, are, in fact, probably a defense against depletion. The body retains water in order to hold onto micronutrients—vitamins and minerals that would otherwise be lost in the urine. Puffiness around the eyes, stocking marks at the ankles, or ring marks on the fingers give fair warning of depletion. When these symptoms occur before menstruation, an increase in all the above-mentioned nutrients may prove helpful. I have found that menstrual cramps can be lessened in severity by supplementation of folic acid, B_{12}, and B_6 plus calcium and magnesium for a week before the period is due.

The menstrual cycle of from 24 to 30 days reflects a wide range of health factors in a woman's life and is the best evidence of her hormonal condition. Menstrual irregularity or the absence of menses, even for months at a time, can often be successfully treated with zinc and vitamin A. And related problems, such as lack of sexual secretions, failure to achieve orgasm, and fibrocystic breast disorder are often cleared up as well. Zinc and vitamin A supplementation often help create a healthier hormone balance. Relying on iron alone for any of these problems is simply not enough.

The most tragic underestimate of the importance of depletion in women has occurred, and still does, in the treatment of depression after childbirth, the so-called postpartum depression. Hospital psychiatric wards are filled with too many young mothers suffering from depression accompanied by suicidal tendencies; many have actually been depleted by the nutritional needs of creating new life and then producing a quart of milk a day to nurture the child. And the physical demands of round-the-clock nursing care for the infant and the stress of the changing family relationship and altered lifestyle must also be considered. All these conditions cause a considerable drain on the energy, hormones, and nutrient supply of the young mother.

Conventional explanations for postpartum depression included the idea of letdown from the exhilaration of giving birth, or that the baby took over the center of attention, thus causing depression in the mother. Instead of putting women on nutritional treatment programs they were placed in locked wards. It seems almost inconceivable that doctors could fail to recognize the double nutrient burden placed on women by nine months of pregnancy and the sudden change in hormonal balance after childbirth. I have seen women who were still nutritionally exhausted a full two years after their delivery. Time after time these cases promptly respond to treatment with nutrient supplements and dietary improvement.

In many books on child care and motherhood, I see references to the problems of changing diapers, constant crying, waking up for feedings at all hours of the night. The authors imply that these problems are causes of frustration and depression. The first year of life is a strenuous and hectic time for the parents, but it is also a time of great joy. When a parent talks about climbing the walls in rage or frustration, I would look at his or her nutritional status first and not just to mental conflicts and personality disorders. It would be a good idea, in my opinion, to take a hair sample from young mothers routinely to test for possible mineral deficiencies. Lacking that, a program of supplemental calcium, magnesium, trace minerals, and folic acid seems to me to be necessary to insure the health and the sanity of all concerned.

One of the unfortunate legacies of the Freudian era in psychiatry is the preoccupation with sexual explanations for mental disorders and, conversely, with mental explanations for sexual problems. No one in Freud's time could have guessed the close connection between nutrition and sex. Pasteur's germ theory of disease was still new, and vitamins had yet to be discovered when Freud developed his theory of infantile sexuality as the source of adult personality conflicts. It was not until after World War II that the effects of nutrition on sexual functioning were recognized.

The American prisoners of war who survived the Bataan "Death March" in 1942 were imprisoned for more than three years. In confinement, they suffered the effects of severe malnutrition. Most lost half their normal body weight; those who survived required months of special rehabilitation. Yet the Army physicians who first attended them were surprised that the soldiers were more concerned about their sexual functioning than with their close brush with death from starvation.

The men reported that their inability to maintain an erection was the most depressing aspect of their confinement. After only a month or so of starvation, they found that they were no longer growing whiskers. Their breasts began to enlarge and their gonads shriveled. They ceased to have normal morning erections. Many of them feared the worst: that they were turning into eunuchs.

Happily, within a few weeks after they were given adequate nutritional therapy, all of these conditions were reversed. A few cases of atrophy of the testicles remained but the male hormone, testosterone, now began to do its work. One by one, the men reported that their "morning manhood" had returned.

Studies of the Bataan prisoners present an interesting historical sidelight, one that also advances our understanding of sexual dysfunction beyond the anachronistic theories that emphasize psychic conflicts as opposed to physical and medical factors. Depletion and hormonal imbalance were too obvious to ignore in these cases. It was also found that some symptoms of these prisoners were due to various pollutants that had been released from their bones and fatty tissues during their ordeal. Chief among these was lead. Lead mobilization, which causes toxicity, can be reversed by the use of ample amounts of phosphorus in one's diet. Lead binds with phosphorus much as calcium does, and this takes it back into safekeeping in the bones. In addition, we now know that extra amounts of iron, zinc, and vitamin C can also help prevent lead from interfering with vital functions in the body chemistry.

Recently, Dr. Carl Pfeiffer has demonstrated that lead levels can be lowered in battery plant workers who are exposed to inorganic lead on the job by feeding them extra amounts of zinc and vitamin C. Within six months of treatment workers' blood lead levels dropped by about 50 percent, while they were still exposed to lead on the job. This confirms the fact that our ability to resist a poison is directly related to the adequacy of our nutrition. However, during actual starvation, such as was endured by the men in Bataan, inactive lead, which has been stored in our bones from childhood exposure, is released and can cause symptoms that are worse than the starvation itself.

I have seen a few such cases in my patients on crash diets. In one such case of lead poisoning, the diagnosis was extremely puzzling until I found that the patient had spent an entire summer at age sixteen painting the exterior of his parents' house. Outdoor-type paint was, and is, very high in lead content. It is likely that a poorly trained or careless worker can inhale or ingest excessive amounts of lead while scraping and sanding the surface. My patient was in a major growth spurt at the time. His diet was high in muscle meat and very low in dairy products— in other words, it was high in phosphorus and low in calcium. Hence, ingested lead would combine with phosphorus and be deposited in the bones as a lead phosphate in greater than usual amounts. If he had been getting more calcium in his diet, calcium phosphate would have displaced some of the lead from the bones and caused it to be excreted in the bile or urine, possibly preventing such a large buildup of lead. With all that stored lead in his bones, any time this man undergoes caloric or nutrient depletion, or even a high-protein diet, lead is released from his bones and causes toxic symptoms: headache, insomnia, aches and pains, and depression.

Lead poisoning is not rare and should not be ignored, but it usually is. Because tetraethyl lead from gasoline is fat soluble and is able to penetrate the blood-brain barrier to damage the brain without leaving a measurable trace in the blood or soft tissue, the diagnosis is usually overlooked or discounted. Also, our medical schools and textbooks teach about clear-cut illnesses, which is to say, advanced and heavy poisoning in which the classic signs are recognizable: anemia, weakness of the long nerves, colic, and mental confusion. Fortunately, most cases of lead poisoning in adults fall short of that. Bodily aches and pains, disturbed sleep, and mental dullness are the most common and distressing symptoms that I have found in patients who have high lead levels. The severity of the symptoms depends on the amount and time of exposure to lead and on whether the lead was from paints and inks, which goes to the bones and soft tissues for storage, or from gasoline, which goes to the brain and nerve tissues.

Martin S. was in his fifties and so warm and likable that I found it hard to believe that he was depressed and had been suffering more or less continuously for fifteen years. Muscle pain, poor sleep, restlessness, and inability to concentrate and remember everyday details made life miserable for him.

No one had thought to investigate the possibility of lead toxicity in all those years. Although he had had a hair test for general mineral screening a year before he consulted me and it had measured 90 parts per million, significantly above the normal limit of 15 parts per million, it had been discounted because it was believed to be an external contaminant from a hair-darkening solution containing lead-based dye. However, there have been a number of cases of severe lead intoxication from this source. Furthermore, this man also was exposed to gasoline fumes for many years in his work as a service station owner. Therefore I ordered tests for lead in his blood and urine, despite the fact that he hadn't been working full time in his repair shop or using the lead-based hair treatment for some years. These tests confirmed that he did indeed have a mild but significant case of lead poisoning, the more significant since tissue levels are known to decrease rapidly when the lead exposure is reduced or ended. In other words, the blood level of lead would have been much higher at the time of exposure. Furthermore, he had been taking vitamin C and zinc for the past year as part of his treatment from a previous physician and this undoubtedly reduced his blood lead level even further. It certainly had helped his illness, for he felt his condition had improved by 50 percent after a year of treatment. When he consulted me his urinary output of lead was now normal. Nevertheless, when I gave him penicillamine, a drug that binds lead and carries it out in the urine, and collected another 24-hour urine sample, the amount of lead was almost quadrupled. This proved that the actual amount of lead stored in his body was greater than the amount circulating freely in his blood. It is noteworthy that the penicillamine also aggravated his symptoms.

With the additional therapy of a high-protein diet, higher doses of vitamin C, and extra selenium, he showed slow but steady improvement, although the memory impairment probably will continue to trouble him. You may be interested to know why I prescribed extra selenium. This mineral is actually toxic in its own right and dangerous in doses over 600 micrograms per day. However, selenium forms an insoluble combination with lead, a selenide, that is nontoxic. Hence, the two minerals are less toxic when present together; each can detoxify the other.

While lead poisoning is likely to be diagnosed as depression in adults, in children it is associated with hyperactivity, learning difficulties, and behavior disorders. Children are more vulnerable to lead than are adults because they absorb it about twenty times more readily while they are growing. The period of greatest danger is actually in infancy when they are likely to put things into their mouths. The eating of or craving unnatural foods is called pica, and it is more likely to occur in children who are deficient in minerals, particularly calcium. Rachel Carson's book *Silent Spring* awakened us to the alarming environmental pollution that our civilization has created. The pollution of our environment is particularly clear with regard to lead because we can compare the lead level in the bones of ancient man and the lead content of ancient layers of the Greenland ice sheet with current levels. There was no lead in the Greenland ice sheet until after 1940, and it has increased each year since then. Modern man has about 500 times the amount of lead in his bones as did his ancient counterpart. On the other hand, you may be reassured to know that hair samples taken from American adults and children in the year 1871 showed ten times as much lead as comparison samples taken in 1971.

Lead pipes and lead-based paint must have been even more a problem a century ago than they are today. In fact, since 1971, the occurrence of lead is on the decline in this country. This is a direct result of government surveys that showed alarming frequency of toxic levels of lead in schoolchildren in Chicago in 1966. Legislation was initiated in 1972 to reduce lead in paint and gasoline, our two most pervasive sources. In 1973 the Center for Disease Control initiated a nationwide screening program. Over 40,000 children were tested at 77 centers; only 6.5 percent had elevated lead in their blood. Compare this with the fact that, between 1969 and 1971, 21 screening programs tested almost 350,000 children and found 20 percent to have an excessive amount of lead in their blood.

Remember, when the blood lead level is increased enough to be considered significant by an official government agency, it is high enough to produce measurable impairment in performance. In the past ten years our appreciation of the dangers of lead has caused a big drop in what is considered a toxic level in the blood. As recently as 1970 it was believed that no treatment was required as long as the blood level was below 80 micrograms per 100 milliliters. The current standard has been reduced to 29 micrograms.

The work of Dr. Oliver David has contributed most to our increased respect for the danger of lead toxicity. In 1974 he reported that in a group of hyperactive children, those whose symptoms were caused by something that had been identified had lower lead levels than those who were undiagnosed. The undiagnosed group presumably had more exposure to lead, which does its damage and then disappears from the blood after a few weeks at most unless there is continued exposure. This makes it hard to diagnose.

In 1976 Dr. David reported additional studies that showed that half the hyperactive children for whom there was no diagnosis showed marked improvement after chelation therapy. The average blood lead level in this group was only 29 micrograms per 100 milliliters. The mean blood lead level was 22 micrograms in the other children. I predict that they too would have improved with chelation therapy to remove lead. The evidence is convincing that any lead at all may be enough to interfere with optimal functioning. Lead is highly attracted to sulfur and thus likely to displace the mineral catalysts, such as calcium, magnesium, zinc, and iron, from sulfur-containing enzymes. This reduces the activity of key enzymes in the nervous system and vital organs.

I want to append a personal testimonial to the value of the hair test in detecting lead exposure. Hair has been used to measure toxic metals, such as lead, mercury, and arsenic, for many years. The murder of Napoleon was proved by means of this test. A lock of his hair revealed the nature of his fate, arsenic poisoning. The diagnosis was possible over a hundred years after his death because hair does not rot very easily and the metals are permanently bound to the structure of the hair.

I was one of the first physicians in clinical practice to begin using the hair test for the other minerals, the nontoxic ones. Therefore I was faced with a problem of obtaining sufficient data for standards against which to compare my patients' test results. I did not fully trust the data base available at that time from the laboratories, especially not in the case of children. It was all too new. Since my wife had given birth to a boy at about that same time, 1971, I impatiently awaited the day when he would have enough hair to test. It took a year! What beautiful red hair it was. But when the results came back from the laboratory I was shocked. The report indicated that at age 13 months our little boy was already suffering from lead poisoning. He had 71 parts per million. Normal for that age—zero.

His blood lead level, when measured a few weeks later, registered only 26 micrograms per 100 milliliters. The source of the lead was found after a lot of detective work. He was not exposed to air pollution or to paint chips from our house. It was a wooden toy, a version of Noah and his Ark that a friend had given my wife. The toy was from Czechoslovakia and had a coat of shiny yellow enamel on Noah's hat. The hat was shaped like a nipple, and my son enjoyed chewing on it. Unfortunately the yellow paint was 6 percent lead—60,000 parts per million. The 1973 legislation set a limit of 5,000 parts per million—it should be even lower.

What a stroke of luck that I had followed my own path in medicine. The hair test no doubt saved my son from becoming a damaged child. With careful attention to diet and supplements of vitamin C and minerals, he has developed completely free of symptoms. He is one of the best students in his class and has enough attention span to be learning a second language and performing in a singing group without noticeable hyperactivity. The sad fact also is that he was unreasonably irritable between ages fourteen and twenty months and had a spell of bowel trouble that required medical consultation before I realized it was due to the lead.

I would be very pleased if those of you with children would mention this to your pediatrician and request that a hair sample be taken twice a year for your children under age 5 as a painless and inexpensive safeguard against this pollutant. Our technological civilization releases 4 million tons of lead per year into the air, and it comes down to the ground in dust. Little children always put their hands in their mouths. The lead content of dirt samples taken from streets in Washington, D.C., has been measured at up to 12,000 parts per million lead! Better keep those hands clean.

The major danger to children, however, will be house paint for a long time to come. Lead-containing paint is chipping off the walls of millions of homes right now. Don't let your children chew on it. Finally, although lead has been removed from pencils, bright-colored ink, which still contains lead that is used in magazines and newspapers, attracts inquisitive toddlers. Protect your child from this hazard and you will decrease the chances that he or she will become hyperactive and will give him a better chance of above-average performance in school. Orthomolecular nutrition and supplements make the odds even better. Studies of prisoners in 1971 and 1973 in two prisons in Switzerland showed blood levels about 40 micrograms per 100 milliliters. A comparison group of blood donors and another of policemen both averaged only half that in the same country.

It takes good luck or a high degree of suspicion to diagnose toxic metal poisoning; the same goes for any chronic poisoning. When more physicians share the orthomolecular approach, I am sure that we will miss fewer cases of pesticide poisoning and fluoride toxicity (from our fluoridated water) than we do now. Just because more cases are not reported doesn't mean they don't exist. It just means that we aren't well prepared to recognize them.

One of the reasons I was receptive to the possibility that nutritional and orthomolecular factors could be important in psychiatry and medicine was that I had so many cases in which patients seemed cooperative and responsive to psychotherapy and hypnosis but still did not feel better or function up to their potential. I realized some other factor must be responsible, and once I began to use the hair test, I quickly learned how valuable it could be to screen my patients for heavy metal poisons, such as mercury.

Bob A. was a forty-eight-year-old dentist who shared my interest in hypnosis. He referred himself for consultation because he was becoming sexually unresponsive, and it was depressing him. At first I thought he had a typical middle-age crisis: his marriage of 25 years had recently ended and he was under pressure to perform with some very lovely women, all of them quite a bit younger. His problem was not only embarrassing to him, it was also heartbreaking, for he was about to lose a lady over it. After two months of weekly hypnosis in which every source of anxiety was reviewed and every positive suggestion was reinforced, we succeeded only in concluding that he might be "trying too hard." His erections, which were not firm to begin with, wilted more as the likelihood of failure drew near. Therapy wasn't helping. No wonder he terminated it after three months.

A year later he returned to give it another try. He was now living with the "love of his life" and was more than ever anxious to please her. In the meantime, I had become involved in the orthomolecular approach. I was now prepared to investigate the medical and nutritional factors that I had failed to appreciate before. I did a hair test: mercury was elevated tenfold and fluoride was increased fivefold above the upper limits of normal.

One of the hazards of being a dentist is the exposure to mercury, which is present in dental amalgam. When the dentist's drill bites into old silver fillings an aerosol effect puts some of that mercury into the room air. This is not dangerous to the patient because it takes multiple exposures at higher doses to accumulate. Nevertheless the hair test is so sensitive that it will usually show a rise of 1 or 2 parts per million after a single visit to the dentist. Normally mercury is less than 1 part per million in hair. In severe poisoning it may rise as high as 600 parts per million. In Bob's case it was only 20 parts per million, not enough to account for his illnesses and impotency but certainly enough to aggravate his symptoms.

I began a comprehensive orthomolecular supplement program with special emphasis on manganese, zinc, calcium, magnesium, and the amino acid methionine. Methionine contains sulfur and is known to remove mercury and lead. I recommended a high-protein diet and vitamin C to further promote the natural chelation and removal of mercury. I hoped the calcium and magnesium would counteract the excess fluoride he had accumulated. Whatever the precise problems were—with so many possibilities it is hard to know for sure—the results were quite clear. His blood pressure dropped to normal within the month and after four months another hair test showed that the mercury level had dropped from 20 to 4 parts per million. He also felt amazingly well and reported, happily, that he didn't need further therapy.

I didn't hear from Bob for a year. Presumably all was going well. Then a note arrived by mail. The stationery was perfumed and the handwriting was graceful and feminine. It was a happy note of thanks, announcing wedding plans and ending with a flourish that I shall always cherish: "From the grateful recipient of one of your former patients. P.S. How do you turn him off?"

It is impossible for me to write about the hazards of environmental and occupational pollutants without being reminded that our worst pollutants—alcohol, tobacco, and mind-altering drugs—are self-inflicted and addictive. I will be brief and practical because I have learned that long and complicated explanations only serve to confuse those salvageable souls who are teetering on the brink of decision regarding their habits. If you want to stop smoking, drinking, or using drugs, I hope that the next few paragraphs will help you to center on your desire for health and success and to sense clearly that addiction can and does interfere with them both. If you do have anything that you really care about, you will find that it is natural to put that ahead of any addiction. It helps to remind yourself: "Addiction is not happiness." On the other hand, there is good evidence that tobacco, alcohol, and drugs are all damaging to health.

Self-Inflicted Pollution

Let me begin with alcohol because it is the least toxic of the three classes of pollutants: alcohol, tobacco and drugs. In fact, alcohol is an orthomolecule: it occurs naturally in the human body. The body even produces an enzyme to convert alcohol to acetaldehyde, which can, in small quantities, be further converted into acetate and used in a number of important ways in the body chemistry. In the form of wine or beer, and particularly ale, alcohol is not only pleasant but also nourishing, particularly in trace minerals. Distilled spirits, however, are far too concentrated for health and contain no beneficial minerals. The most important danger in alcohol is not that it is likely to damage the liver, which it does do after a time, but that it interferes with the nervous system immediately. Loss of mental control due to alcohol is what makes alcoholics: after the first drink they are unable to stop. If you are a problem drinker, no matter how strong your willpower is, it can't be the same after the first drink. Don't try to prove you can be normal, just don't take the first drink.

Alcoholism does run in families and I am impressed by the fact that so many of the patients who have come to me for treatment of alcoholism have had abnormal glucose tolerance tests, particularly showing a diabetic or high sugar level. Mental illness and obesity are also very common in these families. Some of my alcoholic patients have been the most positive responders to nutrient supplements, especially to thiamin, niacin, and B_{15}. I have also been impressed with the relief from cravings for alcohol in some patients when taking glutamine, just as Dr. Roger Williams reported years ago when he proposed that alcoholic humans might reduce their alcohol consumption just as his laboratory rats did, after being fed this amino acid. Other than glucose and ketones, glutamine is the only substance that can be used as a fuel by brain cells. Dr. Williams proposed that alcoholism might result from an impairment in the appetite-regulating mechanism in the hypothalamus of the brain and that glutamine might protect these cells.

Much research must be done before we will settle these questions about the causes of alcoholism. We do know, however, that diabetes does predispose people to alcoholism. According to Dr. Salvatore Lucia, alcoholic beverages were indispensable to the survival of severe diabetics, who were otherwise unable to assimilate enough calories to meet their minimum requirements. Wine is favored by Dr. Lucia because of its slower absorption when taken with a meal.

Do alcoholics differ from nonalcoholics in their metabolism? Two recent studies indicate that they do. In the first of these, a number of alcoholics who developed paralysis of their eye muscles were found to have reduced ability to utilize Vitamin B_1 (thiamin) due to hereditary low levels of the activating enzyme transketolase. In another study, Dr. Marc Schuckit of the University of Washington found that young men with alcoholic parents or siblings had significantly higher concentrations of acetaldehyde in their blood after a dose of alcohol than did a comparable group of men with no familial alcoholism. Both of these studies point to the need for extra amounts of supportive nutrients, such as thiamin, niacinamide and magnesium, if alcoholism is even suspected. It is safe to conclude that if you occasionally drink to excess or if you have an alcohol problem, you can help yourself greatly by careful attention to orthomolecular nutrition and supplements of B vitamins, zinc, and magnesium. But don't use nutrition as a self-justification for heavy drinking: vitamin therapy has failed to prevent cirrhosis of the liver in alcohol-drinking experimental animals.

The latest breakthrough in treating smoking addiction is the use of sodium bicarbonate to alkalinize the blood. A low-protein, high-carbohydrate diet is also reported to be helpful because it is more alkaline. Dr. Stanley Schacter found that an acid condition was associated with a significant increase in smoking. Vegetarians (alkaline) are supposed to abstain; meat eaters (acid), more likely to continue smoking.

I have some reservations about this method because I have had good results with the orthocarbohydrate diet and nutrient supplements, particularly vitamin C and niacinamide, in supporting my patients in the throes of withdrawal from cigarettes. I am more impressed by the patient's degree of commitment to health and to the responsibility of taking good care of the body than to any nutrient factor by itself. My most difficult cases have been in those smokers who regard a cigarette as a "friend." The first step is to see that smoking is an enemy, a very deceptive enemy.

There is always a degree of pleasure in smoking; otherwise no one would smoke. But whatever pleasure smoking may give, it does so at too high a price. Everyone knows about tobacco tars and lung cancer but the advertising now emphasizes low tar and many of you go right on smoking. Keep in mind that smoking also puts other poisons into your system: lead, cadmium, and arsenic all add slowly to the accumulation of toxic metals, while carbon monoxide blatantly snuffs out oxygen with each puff. If you really believe in health you will eventually reject smoking as a personal insult.

Since Dr. Albert Libby and Dr. Irwin Stone reported their promising positive results in treating a series of hard-core narcotics addicts who were able to withdraw from drugs by the use of large doses of ascorbic acid (over 20 grams a day) and a general nutrition program, where all previous means had failed for years before, there have been a number of pilot projects showing that the "natural high" of orthomolecular nutrition is an outstanding contribution to therapy in cases of narcotic addiction.

First Do No Harm

This slogan was presented to the medical profession by Hippocrates, the "Father of Medicine," over 2,000 years ago. It is at the heart of the orthomolecular approach and has attracted many physicians to pursue this "new medicine." Does the new medicine actually work that way? Does the promise of therapeutic safety hold true? Or are we committing nutrient pollution?

Nutrient Pollution?

To my knowledge, there has been no outbreak of nutrition casualties due to overdose, only some well-publicized warnings that it possibly could happen. For instance, Dr. Victor Herbert warned that large doses of vitamin C might cause deficiency in B_{12}. Not a single case of this sort has been discovered and the experiment that Dr. Herbert conducted to demonstrate this has been faulted.

Orthomolecular physicians are all aware of the potential dangers of overdose in treating with fat-soluble vitamins, particularly A and D. However, I feel that reports of the dangers have in general been overemphasized. The toxicity of A is easy to recognize before it reaches the danger stage. Chapped lips and headache are signs that A is building up to excess. It is well established that up to 50,000 units of vitamin

A and 800 units of vitamin D a day are safe and many people can tolerate up to 2,000 units of D. The fat-soluble vitamins E and K are so nontoxic that there is no longer any debate on the subject. I have seen one case of diarrhea for half a day after a single dose of 6,000 units of vitamin E. Vitamin K administration is safe except for patients on anticoagulant therapy because it will inactivate anticoagulants, which could be a hazard.

Vitamin C is also supposed to cause kidney stones. I have not seen a single case in treating several thousands of patients, nor have I heard of one from any of my colleagues in orthomolecular medicine. However, patients who have had an intestinal by-pass operation for obesity excrete increased amounts of oxalates, and the addition of megadose vitamin C might aggravate the situation enough to form stones. The administration of extra magnesium, which competes with calcium to form soluble oxalate, can prevent the formation of actual stones.

No toxicity has been reported with the use of vitamin B_2 (riboflavin), B_{12}, folic acid, or pantothenic acid. There has been no report of toxicity to the use of vitamin B_1 (thiamine) when taken by mouth. Allergic reactions have been observed after intravenous injection, however. Vitamin B_6 (pyridoxine) withdrawal has been observed after abrupt cessation of a 200-milligram dose after a month. There is no known toxicity to biotin. Niacin causes skin flush at low doses and skin rashes at high doses. It also can cause enough stomach irritation that it must be stopped.

Calcium is known to be dangerous in amounts over 3 grams per day. Calcification of the kidneys is the most serious consequence. Magnesium is nontoxic except in cases of kidney failure. Overdose normally gives fair warning, diarrhea. Manganese can be toxic at doses over 100 milligrams per day. I have seen no toxicity signs in my patients who take up to that amount. I did observe tremor and loss of concentration in a woman who had treated herself with 1,500 milligrams per day for half a year. Her manganese hair level was over 30 times greater than normal and, if she continued her self-treatment, she could have damaged her brain cells, resulting in parkinsonism and loss of mental abilities. Because the bowel controls manganese with a special transport protein, it is resistant to manganese overload. Toxicity has occurred almost exclusively in miners and steelworkers who inhale manganese dust. Copper causes nausea, headache, and diarrhea at doses as low as 90 milligrams per day—I observed these symptoms in one of my patients who overdosed one time. She recovered in two days. There is no doubt that copper can be toxic, but no one knows exactly what the upper limit of safety is. A cautious estimate would be about 20 milligrams per 100 pounds of body weight. Zinc has been used safely in children at doses up to 44 milligrams per day and in adults up to 150 milligrams for six months at a time without hazard. However, reduction in copper has recently been reported in adults at about this dose. I recommend that long-term zinc supplements be limited to no more than 60 milligrams per day. Iron is unlikely to be toxic when kept under 100 milligrams per day. However, acute overdose is a danger to children up to age four, who occasionally ingest the contents of a whole bottle. About one death per month happens this way. Selenium is suspect in doses over 300 micrograms per day in adults. Nausea, vomiting, metallic taste, dizziness, and an odor of garlic on the breath are seen in chronic overdose. In children under age five, I suggest that no more than 50 micrograms per day be supplemented. Chromium supplementation is safe up to 1,500 micrograms extra per day. Iodine is known to cause iodism when taken in doses over 40 milligrams per day for more than a few months; headache, severe acne, metallic taste, runny nose, and edema of the lungs may occur. In addition, a low thyroid activity may occur. Acne may be aggravated by iodine at very small doses, as low as a tenth of a milligram per day. Keep this in mind if your skin breaks out after taking vitamin supplements containing iodine.

In summary, there are some real dangers of overdosage from vitamin and mineral substances. However, the same can be said for an overdose of water toxication. The message of orthomolecular medicine is to find your optimal dose. Not too much and not too little.

The difference between nutrient therapy and drug therapy is that one is equally likely to be harmed by too little as too much of a nutrient. It is unlikely that you will ever get sick from a deficiency of any drug. Has anyone ever died of aspirin deficiency? Certainly no one is schizophrenic because of a deficiency of phenothiazine. On the other hand, it is estimated that half of all hospital admissions are a result of adverse effects of drugs. Among my new patients this estimate would be low. The majority of those who come to me on medication exhibit some undesirable side effects.

Dr. Bernard Rimland coined the term "toximolecular therapy" to replace "drug therapy." Drugs are relatively toxic molecules and, though there is much that is good in our modern pharmacology, we must put nutrition—orthomolecular therapy—first.

Toximolecular Pollution

The most toximolecular drugs I know are those that are in common use for the treatment of schizophrenia: the antipsychotic drugs. I do not deny their value. Properly prescribed, they calm the agitated patient and speed up recovery. Furthermore, they can help to prevent relapse and repeated hospitalizations. However, all the drugs of this class, the phenothiazines and butyrophenones, also cause unpleasant side effects, such as dry mouth, stuffy nose, blurred vision, and various muscle symptoms, such as tremor, stiffness, involuntary spasms of the eyes, jaw, neck, or extremities and, worst of all, an incessant feeling of restlessness that keeps the patient in constant motion. No wonder that two out of three patients eventually stop taking the medication.

These symptoms are not entirely unwelcome, for their appearance is an indication that the drug is doing its job—blocking the dopamine neurons in the subcortical areas of the brain that control movement and emotions. There is evidence that the drugs may work by stimulating increased dopamine production in the cortex of the brain itself, and this might be how the drug clears up the disturbed thought patterns so effectively in some patients. However, after as little as a few weeks, the brain cells try to compensate for this blockade by sprouting new terminals and increasing the output of dopamine. The drug must be adjusted to compensate for this.

If all goes well, the patient recovers and eventually stops taking the drug. But, since schizophrenia is often a chronic disease, there is considerable pressure to stay on the drug indefinitely. Unfortunately, we now know that a large number of patients will eventually develop a tardive dyskinesia, a prolonged and sometimes permanent tremor of either the face, jaw, and tongue or the extremities—or both. Because of the facial grimacing and tongue thrusting in dyskinesia, it is also called the "rabbit syndrome."

At the present time, the occurrence of these symptoms is a strong indication to reduce or stop the drug because otherwise the dyskinesia can only get worse. Unfortunately, stopping the drug is not so easy. As the dose is reduced, the movements usually do get worse. Muscle spasms and continuous movements of the face, jaw, and tongue create a hellish picture of what we imagine as madness. Relapse of psychosis is unfortunately common after a month or so, due to release of the emotional centers that have previously been sedated. Now they react with exquisite sensitivity: every fear, every frustration, every suspicion becomes overwhelming. In the worst cases there isn't much that can be done except to resume the medication, increase the dose, and hope that the dosage can be raised enough to stay ahead of the patient's symptoms.

Fortunately, orthomolecular principles have given us some hope for the treatment and prevention of this disorder. When I started out in orthomolecular psychiatry, I had to do a lot of studying on my own. There were no textbooks or journals of orthomolecular medicine, so I began to read medical journals and glean scraps of information from nutrition books. Because of my interest in the hair test and the role of minerals in the functioning of the brain and nervous system, I was particularly alert to information in that field. So it was that I noticed a single line in a review article by the late Dr. George Cotzias, whose pioneering efforts made orthomolecular treatment with L-Dopa available to thousands of victims of Parkinson's disease. Since L-Dopa is an amino acid normally present in the brain, it qualifies as an orthomolecule.

The words that caught my eye read: "phenothiazines chelate manganese." I knew that chelation is an electromagnetic attraction between an organic molecule and a metal ion, so I could suddenly visualize managese getting stuck to these drugs and thus inactivated and removed from physiological activity in the brain.

I also knew from the article that manganese was concentrated in the subcortex of the brain, in those areas that control movement, and that disorders of movement, parkinsonism, could be caused by manganese imbalance. I put two and two together and figured that manganese supplements might correct some of the movement disorder in phenothiazine-treated patients. My theory has proved to be correct. Since 1973 I have treated over 43 cases with outstanding results. In more than half of my cases of tremor of the extremities, symptoms cleared up within a day of taking 30 to 60 milligrams of manganese citrate, chelate, or gluconate per day. I have treated fewer cases of "rabbit syndrome," but of these all have derived at least some benefit from manganese and half have reported greater benefit from niacin. A dose of niacin that is built up enough to suppress the skin flush response works best, usually above 400 milligrams, two or three times per day. In 1975 I reported my first 15 cases in the *Journal of Orthomolecular Psychiatry* and in 1978 I was invited to review my work at the World Congress of Biological Psychiatry in Barcelona, Spain. A number of my colleagues have confirmed that they are getting similar results with manganese and niacin in the treatment of these unfortunate cases of drug-induced movement disorders.

Through the guidance of my colleague, Dr. Carl Pfeiffer, who is an authority on the workings of manganese in the chemistry of the brain, I learned that manganese is involved in the release of acetylcholine, a transmitter substance in the brain responsible for modulating the activity in muscles and in the parasympathetic nervous system. Manganese is also a catalyst for the manufacture of acetylcholine from choline and acetate. I was therefore not surprised when, in 1976, Dr. Leo Hollister of the Palo Alto Veterans Hospital and Dr. Richard Wurtman at the Massachusetts Institute of Technology demonstrated success in treating the "rabbit syndrome" with both lecithin and choline. Though they denied any relation between their treatment and orthomolecular therapy, there is no doubt that both choline and lecithin are molecules normally present in the human body. Furthermore, the doses that they used qualify under the heading "megadose"—up to 15 grams of choline and 6 tablespoonsful of lecithin per day. I think it says something about our progress in orthomolecular medicine when we now have an orthomolecular treatment for a toximolecular problem!

Compared to the dangers of the antipsychotic drugs, the "minor tranquilizers" and barbiturates are relatively harmless although they are more widespread. They do cause addiction and withdrawal symptoms, but the magnitude of the symptoms is less troublesome and the withdrawal always clears up completely.

Nevertheless, I am often asked about how to reduce the doses of these drugs or replace them with foods or nutrient supplements. Here are some suggestions to help reduce "tranquilizer pollution."

When a mild tranquilizer or sedative is needed, start with the simplest of remedies, warm milk, which contains the natural tranquilizer tryptophan. The effect can be further magnified by taking half a glass of orange or grape juice one or two hours later. Juice stimulates the secretion of insulin, which transports tryptophan into the brain. There it is converted into a sedative neurotransmitter, serotonin. Lecithin can be very calming also and may be added to the milk for additional benefits. Inositol, contained in lecithin, may be taken separately in a dose of 1 or 2 grams. Likewise, tryptophan is also available in capsules; a measured dose of 1 to 2 grams may be useful. The ultimate in tranquilizing foods in my experience is calves' brains. A serving of this delicacy with scrambled eggs is high in cholesterol, high in lecithin, and highly relaxing. You may be wondering why I would suggest such a dietary extreme. To my mind, the absence of variety, without an occasional extreme, *is* extreme.

If you still have insomnia, there is another alternative to sedatives: exercise. Vigorous exercise causes the release of hormones called prostaglandins throughout the body. The more you exercise the more your body will discharge them. They promote sleep about 12 hours later. The formula therefore is to have a good run in the morning, eat well and enjoy your day, and increase your chances of a restful sleep at night.

The Nutrition Prescription for Depletion and Pollution

- Follow the principles of orthomolecular nutrition and avoid depletion
- Use nutrient supplements to insure adequacy of micronutrients and prevent depletion
- Remember to increase your supplements at the first sign of illness or when you recognize that you are under stress
- In case of environmental pollution, remember that a high-protein diet is protective against most toxins; also large doses of vitamins A, C, E, and minerals zinc and selenium are known to be protective
- On the other hand, don't forget that nutrients in overdose can be harmful
- Finally, don't underestimate the great achievements of medical science and the great good that many drugs can do
- Just remember: orthomolecular comes before toximolecular—give yourself a chance to heal

10
Arthritis: Something Better Than Aspirin?

Periodically we see reports of a promising new drug for the treatment of arthritis. The stocks of several drug companies rise and fall on the strength of research news or clinical trials in this field. Arthritis is an age-old disorder, one of the five or six most devastating medical problems in this country, affecting some fifty million people. While it doesn't kill you, it can make you wish you were dead.

Arthritis means, literally, inflammation of a joint. Three major types are known: osteo, or degenerative, arthritis; rheumatoid, or inflammatory, arthritis; and gout. The causes of degenerative and inflammatory forms of arthritis are multiple, and the cures are elusive.

By and large, only two classes of treatment are in general use: aspirin and related drugs to relieve pain and reduce swelling and inflammation by reducing the activity of inflammatory substances in the tissues, and cortisone-type hormones that also reduce inflammation but by direct action on the cells in the joints. Gout, which is known to be caused by excesses of a waste product, uric acid, deposited in joints, is treated by diet and drugs, which lower the amount of uric acid. Other than this, however, diet is commonly considered ineffective and not relevant in treating arthritis.

However, in my practice I have seen excellent results from the treatment of arthritis as a mineral imbalance, an allergy, or a vitamin deficiency. All of the treatments are based on nutrient supplementation and dietary manipulation.

The Scenario: The Wrong Minerals in the Wrong Places

Here is an oversimplified description of the development of arthritis due to trauma or wear and tear. Suppose on the first day of your long-awaited vacation you arrive at the airport and enter the terminal. You've decided to carry your bags on board to save time at your destination. It's a long walk to the boarding gate but, in the excitement, you don't notice the weight of the bags.

Next day, however, you find yourself unable to carry the same bags. Now your whole shoulder is tender at rest and downright painful if you dare to lift anything. When you get back home a week later, the shoulder still hurts. An X ray of your shoulder shows calcium deposits in the deltoid bursa, a tiny fluid-filled pouch that normally lubricates the pressure point where the tendon of the deltoid muscle passes over the edge of the shoulder, the acromion. Since calcium crystals are sharp, every movement now causes irritation and pain.

Calcium tends to deposit wherever there is inflammation. It seems likely that tissues subjected to wear and tear undergo increased cellular activity. Lactic acid is a by-product of this increased cell chemistry and, thus, the local tissues become temporarily more acid. Adjacent areas are therefore less acid, and calcium is deposited in these alkaline tissues surrounding the area of inflammation. The reason for this may be simply that calcium phosphate is more soluble in acid than in alkaline fluids; hence it will dissolve in the area of inflammation and precipitate out in the more alkaline surrounding tissues. The closer the site of inflammation is to a source of calcium phosphate, such as bone, the more calcium phosphate is going to be dissolved out of one site and redeposited in another. The amount of calcium phosphate that deposits in a bursa is usually small. In the joint itself rather large amounts of calcium may be deposited, enough to produce deformity in the contour of the bone. After a time the joints are distorted, giving rise to the gnarled, knobby shape that is symptomatic of arthritis. I have observed that magnesium substances can protect against calcium deposits. I will suggest why later.

Areas of wear and tear also seem to concentrate by-products of systemic bacterial or viral infection. Noninfectious materials also concentrate and promote inflammation in our joints by a similar mechanism: allergy. It seems that the weight of our body and friction of movement wear on our joints and normally produce some degree of inflammation. If this coincides with systemic inflammation due to infection or allergy elsewhere in the body, particularly if large numbers of antibody-carrying white blood cells are circulating in their search-and-destroy mission against foreign substances, it seems that some of these may become attracted to and attached in the inflamed joint tissues. These then become sensitized for large numbers of substances. The well-known orthomolecular allergist Dr. Marshall Mandell reports that sublingual allergy tests provoke symptoms of arthritis in over 90 percent of the arthritis patients he has tested. This certainly confirms the experience of Dr. Collin Dong, whose book *The Arthritic's Cookbook* on dietary treatment of arthritis is based upon his successful self-treatment for arthritis, which he found to be due to food allergy. His simple dietary prescription—fish, brown rice, and fresh vegetables—has worked well for thousands of arthritis sufferers over the years.

So, there is a lot that orthomolecular medicine can do to help arthritis sufferers besides advocating aspirin or cortisone. Recently, Dr. John Sorensen has discovered that, by combining aspirin with copper, the resulting copper aspirinate has cortisonelike activity. Whereas aspirin has only 6 percent of the anti-inflammatory activity of cortisone, aspirinate rates 130 percent as active. In addition, when aspirin is combined with copper it no longer irritates the stomach. In fact, it becomes a substance that helps ulcers to heal! Copper aspirinate is an example of a promising new direction in medicine: the combination of a drug molecule not naturally occurring in the body with a vital mineral that plays a natural role in our body chemistry. Undoubtedly, many more such examples will be forthcoming as our knowledge advances and as scientists look into natural mechanisms of our cells and tissues.

Copper, for instance, is clearly involved in tissue repair. It is known to be essential to support energy production in all of our cells but, more important, it is required for the conversion of vitamin C into its two active forms, ascorbic acid and dehydro-ascorbic acid. In the latter case copper is essential to remove a hydrogen ion from ascorbate, and the ion is then used in the manufacture of collagen, the basic protein out of which all our tissues, including bone, cartilage, tendon, and ligament, are made. Iron is also required for the manufacture of collagen; once formed, copper is again required for cross-linking the collagen strands to provide maximum strength and elasticity.

With this in mind it is not difficult to see that imbalances in vitamin C, iron, and copper might be associated with failure to repair wear and tear in the joints. And so it is well known that arthritis can be greatly relieved by giving adequate amounts of vitamin C. It is not as well known that it can be affected by treating with histidine, a naturally occurring amino acid, which binds to copper and zinc. Other amino acid substances that bind to copper, such as penicillamine, have also been successful in treating arthritis. Recently a copper- and zinc-containing protein, orgotein, has been found to reduce arthritis inflammation in horses.

Since metals can be absorbed right through the skin, the fact that so many arthritis sufferers report benefits after wearing a copper bracelet is not so farfetched. There is good evidence that copper absorbed from uterine implants also stimulates production of a hormone, prostaglandin, which has anti-inflammatory effects as well as stimulates growth in young animals. While there is much to be learned about these things, we already have many hints that can guide our efforts to obtain relief from suffering. Niacin, at a dose just sufficient to cause a skin flush reaction (about 100 to 200 milligrams), also relieves arthritis in some cases.

Vitamin A and zinc, which are essential to cellular healing, are also essential in the repair of the inflamed and damaged tissues of arthritis. Dr. Carl Reich has reported moderate to excellent improvement in over half of 300 cases of inflammatory arthritis and in over half of 1,000 cases of osteoarthritis, both types improving with vitamin A treatment alone. In combination with other essential nutrients the results are even better.

Magnesium salts are generally about ten times more soluble than calcium salts, including calcium phosphate. Thus, the presence of magnesium phosphate molecules in the tissues may compete with and interfere with formation of large, insoluble calcium phosphate crystals. By a similar mechanism magnesium protects against the formation of calcium phosphate and oxalate crystals in the urine, which, if extensive, can cause kidney stones. Such a simple dietary strategy as taking a magnesium supplement or including magnesium-rich foods, such as green leaves, seeds and nuts, or shellfish, in one's diet can be remarkably effective.

As long ago as 1943 Dr. William Kaufman reported on a large number of arthritic patients who were helped by the use of megadoses of niacinamide, 1,500 milligrams or more per day. And Dr. John Ellis has had much success in treating arthritis with vitamin B_6, possibly because of its stimulating effect on the immune system and its equally stimulating effect on hormones. Recently, Dr. Edith M. Carlisle has reported that silica is essential in the early phases of calcification of bone. Thus, it is not surprising to find that silica treatment is associated with rapid healing of fractures. Arthritic inflammation causes loss of calcium in the adjacent bone. This weakens the bone and thus makes the joint even more vulnerable. Silica can be protective in such cases by enhancing replacement of calcium. One of my own patients showed a dramatic response to this treatment.

Which Way Would You Turn?

Bruce L. developed painful arthritis of his hands at age fifty. Now fifty-six, for the past two years he was frequently unable to work as a carpenter. His illness was considered "mild" rheumatoid; yet he could barely hold a hammer and actually could not button his shirt. He had consulted a leading arthritis clinic and was taking anti-inflammatory drugs, aspirin and Motrin but with insufficient benefits. In fact, in the past month he had developed tendonitis in his shoulder. In desperation he consulted me, hoping that nutritional medicine might work well enough to permit him to hold onto his job.

There was an obvious clue that food allergy was a factor in his illness: it turned out his hands became more swollen and painful whenever he ate beef—but not lamb. In other words, it wasn't the high phosphorus or fat content of meat that was doing harm, since beef and lamb are about the same in these respects, but the specific nature of the proteins that he must have been allergic to. Further confirmation: he had tried Dr. Dong's anti-arthritis diet, and it had helped him to a limited extent.

A more detailed review of his diet showed an excess of milk; he was drinking over a quart a day. I advised him to reduce his intake and switch to raw milk without added vitamin D. I was particularly cautious about his ingesting any synthetic vitamin D, because this food additive forces the body to absorb calcium even when the body chemistry would normally reject further absorption. At low doses, such as the 400 units in a quart of milk, this is not normally a serious threat to health. However, since he worked out of doors most of the time and already had his quota of natural vitamin D from sunlight, I figured that even a small extra dose should be avoided if possible. Furthermore, it is strongly suspected that chronic intake of vitamin D in amounts as little as 800 units per day increases the likelihood of atherosclerosis and heart disease. It's reasonable to suspect that such a dose might be enough to promote calcium resorption from bone and deposition in areas of stress and inflammation.

Bruce's hair test for minerals also showed no contamination or exposure to lead, which is known to aggravate arthritis. However, all his physiological minerals, including calcium, were moderately low, despite his high intake of milk and generous servings of fruits, green vegetables, and whole-wheat bread. On the other hand, there were no nuts, seeds, or beans in his diet; nor were there organ meats. Trace mineral deficiencies could be related to these dietary shortcomings or possibly to some impairment of absorption from the intestinal tract into the blood. Blood tests confirmed a low level of magnesium and borderline zinc. Iron was not tested, unfortunately; it turned out to be very low in a later hair test.

I prescribed an initial orthomolecular nutrient insurance program and was pleased when, after a couple of weeks, he reported less pain and increased energy. He no longer needed his afternoon nap. This suggested that the supplements were, indeed, satisfying a real bodily need.

Next we attempted to arrive at an orthocarbohydrate level; this was to remove stress and spare the depletion of his adrenal hormones that might otherwise be used up in coping with excess sugar and hypoglycemia. He reported that he actually felt better at a zero carbohydrate level! This was a far cry from the 344 grams that had been his previous habit. Eventually he leveled out at 140 grams, where he was quite comfortable.

Titration (a method of gradually increasing doses) with niacin was then carried out. He developed a pronounced skin flush at 100 milligrams that reached a maximum at 400 milligrams and was no longer present at a dose of 1,200 milligrams. This produced such an improvement that he was able to discontinue the Motrin, an anti-inflammatory drug. He reported equal benefits at a 1,500-milligram dose of niacinamide, taken three times a day. He was well for a month, then he developed bowel cramps. Now he observed that, when he had only one bowel movement a day, his hands hurt the next day; but if he had three movements a day he was symptom-free.

Suspecting that he might be able to build up his antibodies and suppress food allergy with a greater dose of vitamin B_6, I suggested that he try increasing doses. This failed. First he felt dizzy at a dose of 100 milligrams twice a day. He tried again, this time at a dose of 500 milligrams;

within hours he had tenderness and swelling in his gums and mucous membranes. It took more than a week to recover from these symptoms.

Allergy was obviously a central issue in his case, so I gave him instructions for the pulse-test method of identifying food allergies. After an initial half-day fast to determine the resting pulse rate in the absence of food intake, foods are eaten singly and the pulse rate is measured before and after. If the pulse rate speeds up more than ten beats per minute over the highest level in the fasting period, this is usually good evidence of allergy. Both beef and coffee produced a significant pulse elevation. Milk did not and neither did lamb.

Bruce improved steadily during all this time. In exploring his "ecology" we even had his water tested, since it came from a well. The water turned out to be unusually acid and therefore rich in dissolved minerals. There was no change in his condition when he drank only spring water for a month and then went back to well water. However, there was a remarkable improvement when, having heard about the benefits of silica, I prescribed a supplement derived from a silica-rich herb, horsetail.

He was so elated after two months of complete freedom from pain and swelling that he began to reduce his nutrient supplements, first to twice-a-day and then to once-a-day doses. Unfortunately, his symptoms recurred, but this time they were easily controlled simply by restoring his vitamin doses. In particular, he once again found that niacinamide was most clearly of benefit. He also noticed that extra amounts of both zinc and manganese gave him a more complete range of motion. He told me he was able to wrangle cattle now, whereas before orthomolecular treatment he had been unable to fold a sheet. You may be interested to know that the hair test follow-up showed significant increases in his physiologic minerals, especially manganese, magnesium, zinc, and iron, all of which had been low at the outset and all of which were at a healthy level after supplementation.

In the light of all the good results that I have seen in treating arthritis according to the orthomolecular approach, I find it anachronistic that so many physicians and psychiatrists still consider the disease only stress-related or due to psychic conflict. Correlations between nutrient deficiencies and inflammation of the joints are too many and too great to be dismissed.

The question of the heavy use of aspirin and cortisone drugs also has to be answered. I well remember two sisters, both with severe rheumatoid arthritis, whom I treated some years ago. The younger of the two responded completely to an orthomolecular program, much like the program of Bruce L. but without the silica. The older sister had been ill longer and had already been treated for a number of years with cortisone. It proved impossible to get her off drugs and to build her up enough so that her own natural body supply of cortisone could rejuvenate. Unfortunately, high doses of hormones tend to suppress the production of this cortisone by the endocrine glands, and so they eventually atrophy, sometimes never to recover. When it comes to pain relief, I much prefer to use natural tranquilizers and pain relievers, such as the amino acid tryptophan, which is now available at health food stores. In addition, as mentioned previously, copper aspirinate often works amazingly well and has none of the toxic effects of aspirin. Finally, if cortisone effects are needed, the yucca plant produces a saponin with similar effects in reducing inflammation and pain in many difficult cases of arthritis.

The Nutrition Prescription for Arthritis

• See your doctor early and catch it before damage or deformity goes very far

• Watch out for excessive aches and pains after exercise, as they may indicate calcium deposition in soft tissues

• A sign of magnesium need is muscle cramps that don't clear up with vitamin E or potassium

• If you develop permanent bumps on bones at the site of injury or pressure, such as at contact points in your shoes, this indicates excessive calcium deposition and therefore the need for extra magnesium

• On the other hand, beware of the lack of calcium in your diet, especially if you are not eating dairy products regularly or if you like a lot of meat, which increases calcium excretion and therefore also increases calcium need

• A combination calcium and magnesium supplement is good preventive medicine for almost everyone, up to 500 milligrams of calcium and 250 milligrams of magnesium or more, depending on the individual circumstances

• In addition, a complete nutrient supplement with ample amounts of vitamin A, B complex, C, E, and minerals such as manganese, zinc, copper, iron, and silica can be the best additional insurance against arthritis

• Finally, don't believe anyone who tells you that arthritis is not a nutrition-related disease

11
Intestinal Disorders and the Role of Fiber

A friend of mine with whom I play golf once chided me for being so enthusiastic about the virtues of various vitamins and minerals. "You need C for this and E for that and brewer's yeast and magnesium," he said in mock desperation. "It's getting to be like my golf game; there's so much to think about, no wonder I can't hit the ball straight."

Then I told him about fiber.

In 1973 Dr. Dennis Burkitt introduced the results of his studies of bowel disease in relation to dietary habits, comparing native diets in Africa with the dietary habits of Western civilization. His conclusions came like a bombshell on the medical profession: "Removal of fiber from the diet has had a greater deleterious effect on Western health than any other single change." His report exploded the traditional prescribing habits of doctors. The bland and low-roughage diets that had been in vogue for over 70 years are gone!

Dr. Burkitt found that disorders that we accept as common and almost inevitable here are rarely seen in Africa. Diverticula (defects of the intestinal wall), which afflict over one-third of us after age forty, are almost unknown there. The same for hemorrhoids. Colon cancer, second only to lung cancer in the U.S., is rarely seen there. Varicose veins occur in 10 percent of our population but in less than 1 in 1,000 in

Africa. Obesity is a problem for nearly half of us here but in Africa it is a problem rarely seen in those on native diets. It only becomes common after people move to the cities and adopt the Western diet. Coronary heart disease likewise: in the United States it is responsible for a third of all deaths; in Africa it is extremely rare, but the incidence of this disease is just beginning to increase in the large cities.

Naturally, there has been some grumbling about fiber as a cure-all, a panacea. What other single health factor promises benefits in so many conditions: constipation, hemorrhoids, diverticulosis, diverticulitis, varicose veins, hiatal hernia, duodenal ulcers, appendicitis, gallstones, colon cancer, coronary heart disease, and diabetes, to name a few!

I find the story of fiber most interesting because it is an example of the value of clinical rather than laboratory research. This has been the basis of almost all orthomolecular medical progress.

For instance, Dr. A. J. M. Brodribb followed up on Dr. Burkitt's report and studied 40 patients with diverticula. He found that, when compared with people of the same age and sex, these diverticulitis patients had actually only half as much fiber in their diet. They also suffered double the frequency of hemorrhoids and varicose veins, four times the frequency of hiatal hernia and inguinal hernia, and also gallstones. The frequency of appendectomy was doubled.

When treated with two tablespoonsful of wheat bran per day for six months, more than three out of four of these patients showed great improvement. Most interesting was the observation that bowel transit time became faster in patients whose initial transit time was two and a half days or more but it slowed down in those whose initial times were less than a day and a half. In addition, bran thickened liquid stools and softened hard stools—it had a normalizing effect. The bulk weight of the stools increased by almost 50 percent to an average of 90 grams a day, still considerably less than the 200 to 400 grams typical in Africa.

Why Should the Indigestible Part of Food Be So Important?

Fiber increases the size of the stools, as we have already seen. It may be that the simple increase in bulk is what speeds bowel transit time. But what is the source of the increased size of the stools? Is it only the extra fiber? The answer is that the flora, the bacteria that live in the human intestine, are able to reproduce and multiply more rapidly in the presence of fiber. In particular, unprocessed bran flakes provide an increased surface area for the bacteria to grow on. The flakes also spread out and lower the density of the stool, thus allowing water to penetrate and provide better conditions for the aerobic, oxygen-dependent flora to thrive and reproduce. It may surprise you to know that 90 percent of the bulk of our stools is bacteria and that undigested food and fiber normally make up very little bulk. Since the bacteria in our stools actually outnumber the rest of the cells in our body, we are faced with the surprising realization that most of the cells within our body are not our own!

Therefore, the bacteria that we carry in our intestinal tract have a very important impact on our health. This is particularly true because these microorganisms actually complete the digestion of some of our food, producing gases which are absorbed into the bloodstream. In particular the normal intestinal bacteria, the Lactobacillus species, produce harmless carbon dioxide and water. Lactobacillus bacteria also manufacture vitamins, such as vitamin K, biotin, and other B vitamins, in such abundance that they may be our most reliable source of these nutrients—even more reliable than vitamin pills. No wonder then that wherever civilizations include cultured milk products made with Lactobacillus (also called acidophilus) their people are noted for their vitality and longevity.

The presence of fiber clearly favors the growth of healthy intestinal flora, and the increased bulk of the stools stimulates peristalsis, the muscular action of the gut. This propels the fecal contents more rapidly, thus preventing absorption of toxins, reducing irritation of the bowel by carcinogenic bile acids, and promoting the sense of well-being that accompanies healthy functioning.

Since the presence of fiber favors the growth of aerobic bacteria, such as acidophilus, as opposed to anaerobic types that often produce irritating and toxic waste products, this may protect against colon cancer. It is known that anaerobic bacteria digest substances in bile and convert them into carcinogens. The high-fat, low-fiber diet typical of the average American produces sufficient amounts of these irritating substances to cause chronic colitis, diverticula, hemorrhoids, and, eventually, cancer.

So, it seems that not only does fiber encourage the growth of healthy bacteria that produce extra amounts of several important vitamins to improve our health, but also, by permitting water and oxygen to penetrate and mix thoroughly with the soft moist stool, fiber discourages the growth of potentially poisonous and irritating bacteria. In addition fruit and vegetable fibers contain pectin and lignin, substances that are absorbent enough to hold and remove positively charged ions, such as lead, as well as fats and cholesterol.

In Nathan Pritikin's 10 percent fat, 80 percent complex carbohydrate diet, it's quite likely that the absorptive power of the dietary fiber in the complex carbohydrates enables his subjects to lower their serum cholesterol. Fiber absorbs it and carries it out of the system in the stools.

However, reduction of serum cholesterol may not be the only key to the remarkable improvement of so many of Pritikin's followers. Dr. Tom Bassler, a Southern California pathologist and adviser to Pritikin's Longevity Research Institute, is a strong advocate of the possibility that silicon, another mineral nutrient in fiber, is the real hero. He writes:

We put 900 patients on a program of exercise, high fiber diet, and no smoking, and observed them for one month. Those who were at least 20 percent above their ideal weight lost an average 13 pounds. Cholesterol decreased 26 percent and triglycerides decreased 35 percent. Of the 38 diabetics on insulin, 15 were off medication at the end of the month. . . . The average patient was able to walk 10 km per day; 85 percent of the hypertensives were off medication, and symptoms of angina and claudication were lessened. The dramatic improvement in most cases suggests that the fiber itself provides some vital nutrient which is needed for the prevention of both arthritis and atherosclerosis. We believe this nutrient is silicon.

Does It All Come Down to Silicon?

Tom Bassler is a rare combination of gadfly, researcher, and concerned physician. As of this writing, he has run more than 110 marathons, and he has become the leading spokesman for the theory that long-distance running, especially of marathon length, confers immunity from heart disease. Unlike other writers on the subject of atherosclerosis and exercise, however, Dr. Bassler holds that the cardiovascular system is strengthened in exercise, not necessarily by the elevation of the pulse rate, but by nutrition! Vigorous exercise requires the intake of certain nutrients, mainly carbohydrates for energy. Carbohydrates include all the major sources of fiber. And the "active" ingredient in fiber is silicon.

In his book *The Whole Life Diet* and in the newsletter he edits for the American Medical Jogger's Association, Dr. Bassler has championed the role of silicon in building connective tissue and thus affecting everything from arthritis to Achilles' tendonitis. This "ground substance," as he calls it, is a nonmetallic mineral that makes up one-quarter of the earth's surface. It is used in the making of steel and other alloys. In its dioxide form, silica is the chief ingredient of sand. The major source of silicon in food, other than bran, is alfalfa; but it is also plentiful in pectin, yeast, and virtually every dietary fiber. It may be that those few fibers that do not seem to offer benefits to the digestive tract are simply low in silicon.

The most important research work on silicon has been done by the late Dr. Klaus Schwarz of the Department of Biological Chemistry of the UCLA School of Medicine. His studies of population groups in western and eastern Finland—one drinking predominantly hard water and the other soft—have singled out silicon (in the hard water) as the major protective factor against heart disease. Other studies have confirmed his observation that low mortality rates are associated with high levels of silicon in drinking water. Because of its yeast content, incidentally, beer is a fairly good source of silicon.

As long ago as 1962, Dr. Edith M. Carlisle showed that silicon-poor diets invariably induced deformities of bones and cartilage in laboratory animals. Pioneer work in this field has also been done by Jacques and Jacqueline Loeper. In the early 1960s they confirmed that the elasticity and impermeability of the connective tissues of arteries are directly related to the amount of silicon in the blood. In 468 subjects, they reported that the difference in serum silicon between normal and atherosclerotic subjects averaged 17 percent. The role of silicon against atherosclerosis is a sort of "first line of defense": it prevents the weakening or damaging of arterial walls, a precondition for the formation of plaques. Autopsy studies have shown that atherosclerotic arteries contain 14 times less silicon than healthy arteries.

How do you know if your level of silicon is adequate? Dr. Bassler says, with a doctor's typical detachment, "When dietary fiber is adequate, the stool floats and exceeds 25 cm in length." That's about ten inches. But since silicon is also present in the "ground substance" of skin, hair, and nails, you can simply examine them for signs of deficiency. The hair test gives a precise reading and is now widely available. If your fingernails tend to break easily or if your skin is noticeably inelastic, a high-fiber diet can improve both conditions in a matter of weeks. All of the degenerative disorders of the bones, joints, and blood vessels may turn out to be, at least in part, silicon-deficiency diseases.

How Do Diverticula and Hemorrhoids Develop?

Remember that connective tissue is made up of collagen. Collagen, as you will recall, is the most common protein in our body, and it requires vitamin C for its manufacture and repair. Of course, other substances are also part of the intricate chemistry of this substance; chief among them are vitamin B_6 and copper. A number of investigators have linked deficiency of B_6 to hemorrhoids. This deficiency is not rare, especially in women taking hormones. In addition, according to the computer diet analysis, a high proportion of my patients have very low levels of copper in their diet. I wouldn't be surprised if copper deficiency plays a more important role than has been heretofore recognized.

Chronic inflammation of the bowel also weakens the connective tissues. If gas pressure in the bowel should then increase, the weakened supporting tissues give way and the mucosa of the bowel is then pushed out alongside the entranceway of the blood vessel that feeds each segment, forming a diverticulum. Since this is a sac with a small opening, it can trap debris and become inflamed and infected. It is easy to understand that bouts of inflammation also cause congestion of the blood vessels and engorgement of the veins. Now, it so happens that the veins that supply the rectum and anus are lacking in valves to protect against the combination of congestion and increased pressure caused by gravity. When we stand or sit erect, a column of blood in our vena cava puts increasing pressure upon the veins in the anal region. If there is any weakening of the connective tissues in the walls of those veins, they will stretch, and once stretched, they will stay that way. Blood flow through dilated veins is slowed and thus clotting and inflammation occur, leading to the development of hemorrhoids.

I find it erroneous to think that hemorrhoids and varicose veins are caused by straining at stool. Nevertheless, lacking an appreciation of the possibility of nutrient deficiencies, conventional medicine has been attached to such mechanical theories for many decades! Likewise, it is ridiculous to think that the passage of roughage in the stools could cause hemorrhoids, as has been believed until recently. In the words of Dr. David Kritchevsky, "Now we know that moist roughage also means 'softage.'"

Is All Fiber the Same?

While all sources of fiber promote increased bulk and soft, moist stools that pass through the intestinal tract more quickly, there is an important difference between cellulose-type fibers, such as are found in bran, and the stringier lignin and powdery pectin that are found in vegetables and fruits. The pectins and lignins are able to bind and remove fats and cholesterol. By preventing reabsorption of these substances, they actually lower the serum levels of both. This probably accounts for the benefits that have recently been reported in coronary heart disease, gallstones, and diabetes. For example, Japanese researchers have found that a plant fiber, glucomannan, derived from the "devil's tongue" plant, is so effective in controlling diabetes that insulin therapy can often be stopped. Dr. Shomei Matsuura reported a case in which blood sugar and cholesterol levels were normal within two weeks, something that had not been accomplished with insulin therapy. Bran and inert cellulose do not have these particular effects. However, rolled oats and various types of beans (legumes) do. Potatoes and root vegetables are also favored sources of fiber.

Is There Any Danger or Disadvantage with Fiber?

"Fiber may stir the gut but it's unlikely to stir the imagination or quicken the pulse. Attendant borborygmi, flatulence, frequent defecation of soft bulky stools and a constant awareness of bowel activity are hardly conducive to a serene state of mind." So wrote Dr. Samuel Vaisrub in an editorial in the *Journal of the American Medical Association*. His description should be fair warning to go easy when changing your dietary habits. Most people experience an increase in gas when they first try adding bran or other fiber to their diet. This is due to changes in the bowel flora; the addition of a tablespoonful of live Lactobacillus culture, ingested at the same time as the bran, is often quite helpful.

Let me also warn you that it is not wise to take bran repeatedly throughout the day on a regular basis for a long period of time, for it can interfere with the absorption of positively charged mineral ions, such as iron and zinc, and can actually induce deficiency if taken to excess. I was first alerted to this when I found low levels of these minerals in the hair analysis of one of my patients, a fifty-three-year-old man, who had been supplementing extensively with minerals on his own for quite some time without much improvement in his chronic mental dullness and fatigue—until we cut back on bran.

Of course, it is also necessary to keep in mind that some of you may be allergic to wheat and hence to bran, which is the husk of the wheat grain. In that case you will need to rely on apple pectin, vegetable fiber, or psyllium seed if you need a dietary fiber supplement, particularly for constipation.

The prudent rule is to limit your bran intake to two tablespoons a day *at only one meal.* In the American diet, it's unlikely that you'll get too much fiber from sources other than bran, and it's not clear if all fiber tends to deplete iron and zinc. Dr. Robert A. Levine summed up the pros and cons of a high-fiber diet this way: "There is a real hazard: excessive fiber intake can lead to the loss of important nutrients—and whether this is long term isn't known."

Does High Fiber Mean Low Fat?

About 10 percent of food energy in both Western and developing countries comes from protein—but after that a vast difference appears. A Westerner gets 58 percent or more of his calories from fats and sugar, against 8 percent in the diet of the developing countries, where the balance comes from fiber-containing starches and complex carbohydrate grains. Such clear-cut dietary differences in fat and fiber invite research on possible correlations with disease, particularly colon cancer.

Is It the High Fat or the Low Fiber?

Between 1890 and 1960 fat consumption in the United States rose less than 20 percent, but it has increased by 15 percent since 1960. Cereal fiber consumption decreased by 90 percent in the same time period, and, despite the fact that consumption of fruit and vegetable fiber increased by 10 percent or so, this source provides less effect on stool size and bowel transit time than does cereal bran. So we see that both may be applicable to the occurrence of our epidemic of degenerative diseases, particularly diabetes, atherosclerosis and bowel cancer. Our fat intake has increased and our fiber has decreased. To make matters more complicated, let me remind you that our sugar intake per capita more than doubled between 1890 and 1960.

Cancer of the colon has a high incidence where diets are rich in animal fats, refined sugar, and white flour, and low in fiber. The cause of cancer of the colon, however, has been linked more to the lack of fiber. Two similar populations of otherwise healthy, middle-aged men were studied by Dr. Bandaru S. Reddy and his associates at the nutrition division of the Naylor Dana Institute for Disease Prevention: a low-risk group in Kuopio, Finland, and a larger group in New York City with a high risk of colon cancer. Risk was defined relative to the incidence of the disease in the general population of the two cities.

The Finnish group was selected for comparison because it is one of the few in which a *high-fat and high-fiber* diet exists simultaneously. The high-risk group in New York had the usual American dietary mix: *high-fat, low-fiber.* The presence of fat in the Finnish diet apparently was negated by the high fiber.

Bile acids are important factors in causing cancer because they are readily converted by certain bacteria in the bowel into carcinogens. They are formed in the liver and excreted in the bile; therefore high levels are caused by a high-fat diet, because bile is secreted to emulsify fat for absorption. In the study mentioned above, both groups of men had similar, high levels of bile acids, but the water-holding properties of fiber helped dilute these acids in the Finnish group and also shortened the time they remained in the colon.

My friend the golfer might well stop me at this point to complain about information overload. Should we all rush out and buy alfalfa pills, flex our fingernails, or put a ruler in the bathroom? No—we must always be cautious of any "magic" formula. Fiber and silicon have long been ignored in the nutritional mix, and it's time to correct the oversight. But they are only part of a complete program.

The Nutrition Prescription for Intestinal Health

• If you're under the care of a doctor for any of the above disorders, ask him about fiber. Most doctors have regained respect for this health-giving, indigestible part of our food

• If you're in good health, start thinking about a gradual shift in your diet to fiber-rich foods. If you're already eating two servings of vegetables and two servings of whole grains (including whole-wheat bread) a day, you're probably getting enough fiber. If you're not, and find it inconvenient to start that sort of a diet, at least add raw bran flakes to your other food. (Not commercial bran cereals but the raw, unprocessed bran you can get at a health food store.) If wheat bran irritates you, then try rice bran, apple pectin, or vegetable fiber instead

• If you have mild, self-treatable chronic problems such as constipation, diarrhea, gas, overweight, or any time you are taking antibiotics, give your fiber a boost with Lactobacillus acidophilus. These health-giving bacteria are available at health food stores in liquid culture or freeze-dried tablets. Cultured milks, such as buttermilk, yogurt, and kefir, are another source but must be pasteurized before, not after, incubation in order to be of benefit. If liquid appears when these milks stand at room temperature for an hour, then the L. acidophilus are alive

• Condition yourself for a lifetime of fiber-consciousness. Eat whole grains, the pulp of fruit, and unrefined root vegetables, especially potatoes and sweet potatoes

• If bowel problems persist, even after all these positive steps, don't overlook the possibility of an undiagnosed intestinal parasite

12
Allergy and Immunity

A recurring theme of orthomolecular medicine is its rediscovery and validation of some of the time-hallowed beliefs of folk medicine. "An apple a day keeps the doctor away" can now be viewed as a case of adding fiber and silicon to your diet. And we have seen that supernutrition through whole foods can lead to increased well-being. Indeed, it now makes some sense that oysters, a rich source of zinc and other minerals, can be especially good for your sex life. In this chapter we will see that grandmother's advice to "starve a fever and feed a cold" was perhaps her most important wisdom about self-treatment at home.

Allergy is an overreaction or even an unnecessary reaction of the body cells to foreign materials. The ability to identify the self (our own genes) from the nonself (anti-gene or antigen) is one of the most essential functions of life. Nature has wisely evolved the immune system, a method of recognizing, remembering, and getting rid of harmful antigens. This is the basis of resistance to infection. It is also the basis of allergy.

Antigen molecules can enter the body through the mouth, the nose, or by direct contact with the skin. Normally, food, water, and air are harmless and do not cause irritation or allergy. However, harmful substances or events that do damage cells also produce a number of chemicals, particularly histamine. The amount of chemicals released conveys the message about the extent of damage to the immune system.

Nature has evolved a few methods of getting rid of almost all nonself substances, either cellular or simply molecular. Special cells in the thymus gland, called T-lymphocytes, are activated by whatever substance they contact that does not fit normally with the receptors on the lymphocyte surface. This causes the lymphocyte to produce antibodies, proteins that stick to the enemy cells or molecules. Antibodies will also coat other cells throughout the body, particularly lymphocytes of another type, the B-lymphocytes. Normally the B-cells are present in small numbers. However, if enemy molecules are very much in abundance, they cause T-cells to produce more antibody, enough to initiate a more pronounced effect as quantities of other cells and substances are stimulated in a chain reaction of defensive actions by the body cells. We recognize this as inflammation: blood vessels dilate and the area turns red and hot from increased blood flow and swollen from the leakage of fluids. If the defensive cells release their lysozymes, chemicals that dissolve cells, some local cells of the body may be demaged—much like full-scale war where planes have to drop bombs on friendly troops as well as on the enemy.

In short, inflammation is the visible sign of the body defenses at work. The system is: recognize, remember, mobilize, and destroy. In the process innocent cells also get damaged. After the battle is over these must be repaired.

The thymus gland, located just below the thyroid at the base of the neck, is known to coordinate the immune response. In particular, T-lymphocytes, derived from the thymus, have receptors on their surface that can interact with histamine. Histamine activates the T-cells to manufacture protein molecules, antibodies, that match the antigens that caused the initial damage. This functions as a permanent memory in the T-cells, which can be transferred to the other cells throughout the body so that a variety of weapons—antibodies, enzymes, or "killer cells" that engulf and remove invaders—can be used to destroy the antigen.

While it takes a few days for T-cells to become sensitized to a new antigen, on re-exposure the response is immediate. The T-cells ingest and digest the antigen but also secrete chemicals that activate a swarm of other cells throughout the body, the B-lymphocytes. This magnifies the immune response and, in particular, increases the amount of antibody available to combine with and target antigen for destruction.

In mild infections without fever, such as a cold, there is less likelihood of releasing enough histamine and other chemicals to activate the T-lymphocytes. Hence it is safe to eat because the food molecules will not be targeted by the activated lymphocytes and the nutrients will hasten recovery. On the other hand, fever is a sign of more intense or general inflammation and higher histamine levels, sufficient to activate the T-cells. Fasting (water or vegetable broth only) during the few days one has a fever can reduce the likelihood of developing allergies to foods. During the period of fever when the T-cells are actively producing antibodies, it is wise to avoid dust and pollens as well, so as to avoid nasal allergy. Allergies are like conditioned reflexes: they form by association—but only at a critical time.

Diet and emotions can strongly influence this process because T-cells respond not only to histamine but also to adrenalin, cortisone, and insulin. Adrenalin and cortisone can inhibit T-cell activity and thus reduce immunity. That is why cortisone should not be taken during infection and why physical or emotional stress that causes release of adrenal hormones interferes with resistance to infection. Insulin, on the other hand, is known to increase the intensity of the T-lymphocytes' response, and thus increases immunity. Lack of insulin, as in diabetes, is associated with diminished ability to resist infection. Excessive insulin secretion, as in hypoglycemia or the excess intake of refined carbohydrates, can increase the inflammatory response in case of infection and can aggravate allergy as well.

Until recently it was not widely appreciated that substances ingested by mouth, such as food, actually do reach the internal organs unaltered. Digestion does not completely break them down. The brain, in particular, was believed to be protected from antigen more than any other organ in the body. In 1882 the great researcher Dr. Paul Ehrlich demonstrated that animals given vital dyes become intensely stained in all parts of the body except the brain. Even when dye was injected directly into the bloodstream the brain of the laboratory rats remained snow white! Therefore, allergy of the brain was considered unlikely.

Recently, however, Dr. W. A. Hemmings at the University College of North Wales has demonstrated that various plant and animal proteins do, indeed, show up in the brain, where they are measurable by radioactive tracer and precipitation with immune sera. Most important, the fragments that were found in the brain retained the antigenic structure of the original molecules.

As long ago as the turn of the century, Dr. P. T. Uhlenhuth reported that after he fed egg whites to rabbits, he could detect antibodies to egg albumin in the blood. Not long after that it was discovered that, if the amount of antibody was stimulated even further by injecting the antigen, then the animals would go into anaphylactic shock when they next ate egg white. The first sign of the shock state was "intoxication," a state of motor uncoordination, which is also a sign of cerebral allergy.

Despite the foregoing, which substantiates the mechanisms of cerebral allergy, I am not convinced that this type of mechanism plays a usual role in producing the symptoms such as headache, dizziness, lightheadedness, irritability, muscle tension or uncoordination, mental dullness, emotional outbursts or even outright paranoia that are so commonly ascribed to cerebral allergy. I am of the opinion that the symptoms of the immune disorders of the brain must take the form of a more prolonged reaction, as in multiple sclerosis, where the spells of disorder last not for hours but for days, weeks, or months.

Cerebral symptoms are indirect by-products of allergy in the body tissues, which release inflammatory hormones, such as histamine, prostaglandins, and a number of others, and provoke discharge of adrenal hormones. In addition, certain mental symptoms come on almost immediately after exposure to specific foods and/or inhalants. These symptoms have been verified many times by orthomolecular allergists, such as Dr. Marshall Mandell and Dr. William Philpott, whose sublingual testing revealed 90 percent occurrence of such allergy in schizophrenia: 64 percent to wheat, 52 percent to corn, 50 percent to milk, and 86 percent to tobacco!

In my own practice I have had ample opportunity to confirm that there is a direct relationship between food and mood. It is commonplace for my patients to report positive as well as negative emotional responses within minutes of ingesting certain foods. Naturally, when this becomes important to diagnosis, the test procedures can be done systematically. Test meals can be planned, one food at a time, or a few drops of extract placed under the tongue. It is a good idea to have plenty of distilled water to drink and sodium ascorbate and sodium-potassium bicarbonate on hand to "clear" allergic symptoms, should they occur.

Most physicians are not prepared to accept the possibility of an immediate cerebral response to small amounts of foods placed under the tongue or of volatile aerosols or hydrocarbons inhaled. However, the anatomical design of the blood-brain barrier itself lends support to the fact that the brain is designed to sample the contents of the blood supply at the first bite of food or the first whiff of air.

There are a few parts of the brain that are not sealed off by a blood-brain barrier—the hypothalamus, pituitary, and pineal. When the rest of the brain remains white after a blue dye is injected into the blood, these nerve centers stain deeply. It makes a lot of sense that these brain centers, which are known to control our responses to chemical substances by affecting our emotions and body rhythms, would be designed to respond to minimal doses of foods or inhalants and regulate the proper emotional-hormonal response to the ingested molecules. Thus, an offensive molecule, an irritant or allergen, can be immediately detected before one ingests enough to do greater harm or trigger off a true inflammatory response. Cerebral allergy is a strong reaction: anxiety, nausea, headache, lethargy, and depressed moods are common. The brain function is clearly impaired, but only temporarily, for tissue destruction is unlikely. Complete recovery from cerebral allergy is the rule.

Is It Possible to Overcome Cerebral Allergy?

Good results are almost always seen when successful avoidance of the allergens is accomplished. Just as your poison-ivy skin rash will clear up when you avoid poison ivy, your asthmatic wheezing due to milk protein will clear after you avoid milk and milk products, and your mental impairment may improve dramatically when you identify the offending allergen molecules and remove them from your environment.

If you cannot achieve total avoidance, it is often possible to achieve good results by simply reducing the amount of exposure to the allergen. I well remember one 50-year-old man whose adult-onset asthma responded so well to orthomolecular nutrient supplementation, de-stressing through the orthocarbohydrate diet, niacin, and partial avoidance of milk and eggs that he was able to stop all medications, including his cortisone inhalers, for the first time in three years. His wheezing would recur if he ate eggs three days in a row. One day he got overconfident and made up a health drink for himself. Instead of the usual half glass of milk he took a full glass, and instead of a teaspoonful of yeast he took a tablespoonful. He learned his lesson: within half an hour his asthma returned full force and he had to visit the emergency room for a shot of adrenalin. Incidentally, he had been troubled by paranoid feelings and thoughts of people plotting to influence him for 30 years. These decreased along with his allergies and were almost gone after the addition of vitamin B_6 to his nutrient supplementation.

Rotation diets are perhaps the most practical way of dealing with food allergies. In these diets, no food substance is eaten more often than once in four days. This assures that there will be no overload of allergen molecules; yet at the same time, continued exposure to at least some of the allergen stimulates the T-cells to activate B-cells, which act as blocking antibodies in the intestinal tract. These blocking antibodies assure that less of the allergen gets through the intestinal barrier. If bowel transit time is rapid, the rotation can be successfully accomplished every three days instead of four.

Fortunately, most patients with allergies are able to suppress allergic symptoms when they are well nourished and not under excessive stress within themselves or from their environments. I have observed that an attitude of optimism not only helps to bear up under unpleasant symptoms but also speeds recovery. After all, your body is designed to heal; therefore, enjoy healing.

Allergen desensitization is another technique that works. Just as the physician may inject minute amounts of antigen to provoke the immune response, hopefully to build up blocking antibodies and suppressor cells that can reduce the inflammatory response to allergy, so can continued exposure to the allergen gradually reduce the allergy. This is treacherous, even dangerous, if you have severe symptoms of allergy, such as asthma or anaphylaxis. However, with milder cases, such as hay fever and skin rashes, regular exposure to small amounts of allergen seem to overcome the allergy—if you are well-nourished.

Desensitization is not likely to work in cases of diarrhea and colitis, however, for in this case the buildup of B-cells in the intestinal wall primes the intestine for more diarrhea and inflammation. Likewise, desensitization is unlikely to work in cerebral allergy. This type of allergy is triggered by absorption of allergen directly from veins of the tongue and palate that go directly to the brain. The buildup of intestinal blocking antibodies can do no good in that case.

Large amounts of certain nutrients can be particularly helpful in overcoming allergies. Vitamin A and zinc work together to increase production of antibodies. Vitamin B_6 and B_{12} and folic acid are also important in antibody formation. Vitamin C and pantothenic acid are vital to the production of adrenal hormones, which have an anti-allergic effect. Recently, Dr. A. Fidanza and his colleagues at the University of Rome demonstrated that, when rats were given a very large dose of pantothenate, the amount of steroid hormones in their adrenal glands doubled in six hours!

The followintg case report from my files shows how a localized irritant, saccharine, and a cerebral allergy to corn sugar and milk can combine to present quite a puzzle for both diagnosis and treatment.

Sonia T. was an attractive, popular college girl. She was overweight—190 pounds—but she carried it well for her height of 5 feet 9 inches. She appeared to me to be a very pleasant young woman. Her mother was convinced she was depressed. Sonia didn't feel well, but she just wasn't the type to complain despite the fact that she had constant burning in her stomach. Her mother urged her to consult me because she had lost her spark, lost interest in her studies and social life.

Her family doctor agreed that she was emotionally disturbed and that psychiatric help was in order. Meantime, he was treating her with antacids and a histamine-blocking drug, Cimetidine.

The computer diet analysis revealed that she had a fairly typical overweight teenager diet: 2,500 calories, half of which came from carbohydrates, mostly refined, but with enough variety in her vegetables so that she was only deficient in nine vitamins and minerals. More important than the actual nutrient levels, it had never occurred to anyone to check the beverages she was drinking—four to six bottles of diet soda per day. Since saccharine is known to be a weak carcinogen, I wondered if it might not also be a direct-contact irritant. I recommended that she drink only water for a few days. She improved in a day and within three days the burning, squeezing pains in her solar plexus were gone. When she resumed diet drinks the pain returned almost at once. She needed no further persuading.

After she had taken nutrient supplements for two weeks, she was still rather lethargic and relatively depressed in mood. The orthocarbohydrate diet, as described in Chapter 15, proved of almost immediate benefit. Her mood improved as she dropped her carbohydrate intake from an initial level of over 300 grams per day to only 30 grams per day, so small an amount that she maintained a state of moderate ketosis. She lost 8 pounds in the first two weeks and was under 160 in three and a half months. She also began to walk and exercise more as her energy level came back. This increased her need for complex carbohydrates, up to 60 grams per day. As her weight loss progressed she told me, "My friends have to remind me to eat, and I eat only when I'm hungry." She also found it helpful to set aside one day a week to go without eating.

Improvement in her state of well-being certainly helped to promote the self-conditioning that she experienced. But the loss of cravings for food in this formerly obese young woman was a tipoff to the removal of allergens, in her case refined carbohydrates, particularly sugar and corn syrup, that had previously irritated her intestinal tract, causing a sensation of craving. At the same time, I believe that some of these same allergens made her both irritable and depressed. I have no other explanation for the rapidity with which her mood and personality functioning improved.

Also, in Sonia's case, ketosis may have had a calming effect on the mood system of her brain, for ketones are known tranquilizers. Recent research had demonstrated that ketones derived from the burning of fat tissue act as a reserve fuel supply when carbohydrates are low in the diet and that the ketones are utilized mostly in the deeper layers of the brain, especially in the emotional-chemical control centers of the pituitary, pineal, and hypothalamus. In cases of allergy or anxiety such as this one, these are exactly the nerve centers that need extra fuel and a tranquilizerlike action.

The Process of Elimination to Discover Allergies

With only a little coaching from an orthomolecular physician or allergist the layperson can go a long way toward identifying molecular "enemies" in foods and in the environment. One would think that most allergies are obvious: sneezing when the pollen count is high, diarrhea after drinking milk, turning red in the face after a few sips of alcohol. In the most serious cases, though, there is a *masking effect* that can completely obscure the source of the affliction.

Investigation in this field was begun by Dr. Albert Rowe, a California allergist, in the 1920s. In the thirties and forties, a Midwestern physician, Dr. Herbert Rinkel, explored the masking effect. Later Dr. Theron Randolph of Northwestern University developed specific techniques to get behind the mask. Their theory is that the body must be cleared of all allergens before a specific reaction to that substance can be singled out. In alcoholism, for example, the craving for drink is explained as a need to assuage withdrawal symptoms from the last drinking bout—in other words, another drink is needed to cure the hangover. But the continued drinking fails to produce any allergic symptoms—they become buried or masked in the following round.

In Dr. Randolph's clinical ecology unit in Zion Benton Hospital near Chicago, patients suffering from a variety of undetermined allergies are carefully screened from the outside world in rooms that are practically sealed off from contamination by air and water pollution. Treatment begins with a distilled water fast of four days or more—until the withdrawal symptoms go away. Withdrawal symptoms that make their appearance at the end of the first day are usually cleared by the fourth.

Then test meals, each consisting of a single well-controlled food, are systematically served. Dr. Randolph has shown that under these conditions, which he calls "detoxifying" the patient, a formerly masked food allergy will produce spectacular symptoms at once.

Here is a case where the pulse test helped my patient recover from skin and cerebral allergy that had made her life miserable since infancy.

Susan C., a twenty-six-year-old artist, had been troubled by generalized eczema since age two. Despite treatment several times a year with antihistamine and cortisone drugs to control flare-ups, she never really was rid of the itchy, scaly, and sometimes open sores on her face, arms, trunk—everywhere. Her skin was markedly thickened, pigmented, and scarred from inflammation, scratching, and application of various chemicals in an attempt to find a cure. Relapses seemed to be caused by frustration and repressed anger that she ordinarily did not recognize until afterward. Anxiety attacks with rapid pulse and overbreathing had occurred every few months at times of family crisis, particularly arguments with her father. Because of her unsightly skin she had little social life and her relationships with her family were overly important.

The computer diet showed 1,800 calories and with carbohydrate intake of 120 grams, of which refined total carbohydrate was only 20 percent. Fat accounted for over half her calories, but there was very little sugar and plenty of beans and Chinese vegetable dishes so that her nutrient intake was deficient in only 8 out of the 26 items computed and at that only about a third to a half below the Recommended Daily Allowance levels. This was a better than usual diet profile among my patients. The blood test found no deficiencies in the several vitamins and minerals that were checked; however, the hair test was low in manganese and zinc and high in mercury, the latter probably due to exposure to mercury-containing skin ointments, such as ammoniated mercury, over the years.

Her skin improved just a little after treatment with vitamin-mineral supplementation, but she also found her mind was clearer. It turned out that she had also been having rather severe mental symptoms along with her eczema for years. These symptoms were typical of schizophrenia (feelings of unreality, visions, mental confusion), yet her personality was really quite pleasant and likable, not alienated, paranoid, and indefinite as is typical of many schizophrenics. The combination of a positive personality with spells of sensory dysperception and mental impairment is typical of cerebral allergy.

After a day's adherence to an almost zero-carbohydrate diet, she produced urinary ketones. As a result, in her case she felt irritable and mentally more "spaced out." In another day, after she added in a bare 15 grams of carbohydrate, she came out of ketosis. The unmasking of allergy became obvious. Her carbohydrate this day was in the form of wheat bread, and she felt "hot all over" within 15 minutes. This was a tipoff to allergy, so I urged her to study her reactions systematically with the Pulse Test method that is included in this chapter on page 167. This procedure demonstrated clearcut pulse elevations to wheat, cheese, almonds, and shrimp, and also to peaches, yogurt, and cat fur.

Susan's skin began clearing up, better than it had in years, after avoidance of these diagnosed allergens. Because she had chronic constipation, I prescribed extra magnesium oxide. When her total magnesium intake reached a gram per day, she developed loose stools.

Then we lowered the dose. This simple treatment acts as a combined gentle laxative, anti-allergen, and mild tranquilizer. By speeding up the bowel transit she was able to rid her body of allergens more quickly.

Susan was doing so well after four months of treatment that we did not expect any further skin improvement. Because her mental symptoms were similar to schizophrenia I decided to try even larger doses of zinc and vitamin B_6. Both her mental symptoms and skin got dramatically better with 30 milligrams of zinc and 500 milligrams of B_6 twice a day. She became truly excited about her improvement: for the first time in years, her hallucinatory visions of spirits, faces, and animals completely disappeared so that she was no longer afraid of the dark. Her mental concentration improved amazingly: she enjoyed reading for the first time in her life. Meantime, her skin improved further and became soft and smooth, losing the scarred and dusky pigment that had concealed her beauty. No wonder her newfound boyfriend proposed. I still get a card from her every Christmas. She has remained well.

I want to briefly describe my experience with another fine young woman whose life had been tragically marred by undiagnosed orthomolecular and allergic problems. Wendy V., twenty-nine, had been troubled by agoraphobia and depression ever since dropping out of college in her senior year eight years before. For three years she was a semi-alcoholic recluse. Psychotherapy helped "somewhat," but she felt greater benefits from reading a book about self-treatment through autosuggestion by Dr. Clare Weeks. In the past three years she improved further

NAME_____ DATE_____

Allergy and food intolerance may be revealed by pulse rate increases. Airborne allergens usually cause pulse increases of less than ten per minute. Food allergens cause increases over ten per minute. The chart below starts with a half-day fast during which your pulse rate is checked every two hours to establish the normal range. The pulse rate is then checked before and after exposure to suspected foods, as charted, or you may adjust according to your own suspicions. To take your pulse accurately: Be seated. Allow a minute of rest. Then place the left index finger against the base of the right thumb and count the pulse beats for 60 seconds. NOTE· After a food has been found to be non-allergenic by the pulse test it may be included at the succeeding test meals.

Pulse	Date Time Waking	FOOD	Pulse	Date Time Waking	FOOD	Pulse	Date Time Waking	FOOD
	8:00 am	FASTING		8:00 am	2 slices bread		8:00 am	20 almonds or walnuts
	8:30 am			8:30 am			8:30 am	
	9:00			9:00			9:00	
	9:30			9:30			9:30	
	10:00 am	FAST		10:00 am	2 eggs		10:00 am	apple
	10:30			10:30			10:30	
	11:00			11:00			11:00	
	11:30			11:30			11:30	
	12:00 pm	FAST		12:00 noon	cheese		12:00 noon	liver
	12:30			12:30			12:30	
	1:00			1:00			1:00	
	1:30			1:30			1:30	
	2:00 pm	FAST		2:00 pm	carrot		2:00 pm	bacon
	2:30			2:30			2:30	
	3:00			3:00			3:00	
	3:30			3:30			3:30	
	4:00 pm	8 oz. milk or yogurt		4:00 pm	orange		4:00 om	potato
	4:30			4:30			4:30	
	5:00			5:00			5:00	
	5:30			5:30			5:30	
	6:00 pm	beef		6:00 pm	fish		6:00 pm	ham
	6:30			6:30			6:30	
	7:00			7:00			7:00	
	7:30			7:30			7:30	

Copyright 1978 Richard A. Kunin

by self-treatment with nutrients and a low-carbohydrate diet. However, fatigue, mood depression, anxiety, lack of confidence, and poor concentration and memory sapped her confidence so as to force social withdrawal. She was suspicious of allergy because she had found that inhalants, such as dog hair, and foods, such as wheat, milk, cheese, citrus, and yeast, all raised her pulse rate. She tested this after reading Dr. Arthur Coca's book (*The Pulse Test*).

Physical examination did not find much: just skin blemishes, particularly around the mouth and chin, and a moderately coated tongue, probably indicative of weak stomach acid. She also had a slightly enlarged thyroid gland. The blood tests were mostly normal; however, the red blood cell count was slightly low, although her vitamins and minerals were normal. Her diet was so low in carbohydrates that urinalysis showed ketones from the outset, before the orthocarbohydrate procedure. Thyroid tests were normal. Serum histamine was slightly elevated. The glucose tolerance test showed normal levels of blood sugar over the five hours of the test; however, she was depressed and weepy two hours into the test, at a time when her sugar level was normal. This probably was due to allergy to the corn syrup in the sugar solution given for the test.

She improved with nutrient therapy, and she realized that she felt much better also because she was avoiding milk and wheat. The orthocarbohydrate diet found her in good spirits in ketosis and at her best at the optimum point of 60 grams. When she increased her carbohydrates to 220 grams, she felt a return of fatigue and dyspepsia. This convinced her once again to discontinue eating milk and wheat.

In the course of her orthomolecular therapy the mineral levels in her hair, all of which had been quite low at the beginning, normalized. I think you will get a better idea of what she went through from her letter of appreciation written to me a year later.

> When I decided to see you, I had already been seeing a psychiatrist and had benefited a great deal. However, I could not understand why my moods and energy were subject to such frequent extremes. Now I feel I am at last in control of these disturbing phenomena, among numerous others.
>
> I originally suspected that I might have some food sensitivities which might be causing some of my problems. (I already discovered that I got headaches and painful aches in my finger joints from soybeans.) My symptoms sounded very similar, especially the fatigue withdrawal syndrome and the various types of irritability and sensitivity. I needed to see you to confirm or deny these suspicions; I was ready to drop them if unfounded,

but I could not drop them without discussing them with an expert who would take them seriously. The very fact that you did take them seriously was a tremendous relief and boost, and it meant that I was able to cut milk products out of my diet assiduously for once, no longer feeling sheepish. Due to this I have lost ten pounds permanently, along with a lot of bloating and indigestion; anxiety has diminished; mental slowness and confusion are gone, along with memory lapses, dreamy states, lethargy and apathy, relatively long periods of crippling depression and rapid mood changes, speech difficulties, the constant frog I had in my throat for a time, most shooting pains and spasms, most spells of irritability and a lot of my anger, resentment and impatience. The skin of my face no longer breaks out.

My obsessions and compulsions have loosened their grip. I have been able to keep a journal without worrying that it is unfinished, and can take notes and read with far less nagging compulsiveness. Also, I no longer have the "hangovers" that I did. I no longer have cravings after eating certain foods. I did very much crave cheese, yogurt, ice cream, starches, etc., the next few days after eating them. I would be exhausted, very depressed and unable to function at any efficient level. I would be unable to even get up till late morning or early afternoon. This is very similar to the hangovers I would have when I abused alcohol. My head would feel gluey and tense inside, I would feel quite guilty, and also extremely inferior and undeserving. The looks of strangers would feel like stabs.

All the above symptoms have reminded me of the numerous symptoms I had as a child—hating to get up, weakness in my hands, "growing pains," spells of dizziness and nausea, frequent spells of gas, etc. The thing that is striking to me is that now I feel I can handle the few symptoms that do occur.

Treating her allergies by avoidance was of the greatest help to her.

Allergens Do Not Always Come from Outside Your Body

Here is a case in which an inadequately treated vaginal monilia made a young woman's life miserable for seven years not only due to vaginal irritation but also depression caused by cerebral allergy to the monilia organisms. Although she was treated on multiple occasions with the best antifungal antibiotics, her vaginal inflammation and discharge recurred. She was so tender from chronic infection that she was afraid to marry. In addition, she found herself subject to physical fatigue, irritability, and depression, a far cry from her usually energetic and outgoing personality. These spells coincided with flare-ups in her infection. When I examined her abdomen it was obvious from the generalized deep tenderness there that she had inflammation in her intestinal tract as well as in her vaginal tissues.

The cause of her prolonged disorder appeared to be a faulty and incomplete vegetarian diet. For years she had been depleted of zinc and vitamin A due to excesses of grains that interfered with mineral absorption and insufficient green and yellow vegetables, which normally are the source of vitamin A, carotene. Stool analysis revealed an overgrowth of monilia, so I treated her fungus vigorously with antibiotic tablets taken by mouth as well as by vaginal suppository. I also prescribed acidophilus culture to help displace the fungus with health-giving bacteria. Finally, the orthomolecular nutrition program was designed to support resistance to infection and tissue repair: high doses of vitamin A and C plus extra amounts of zinc and manganese, in particular.

This time she made a complete recovery from the monilia. As expected, her depression lifted promptly, as soon as the source of monilia antigen was removed from her system.

Complete avoidance of allergens is not always necessary. Some people have the ability to suppress allergy symptoms so that, while the allergy still exists, the symptoms are hardly noticeable. At times of stress, fatigue, or nutritional imbalance, however, symptoms may return.

Donald D., a thirty-one-year-old executive, was very concerned about bloody diarrhea that he had been unable to cure in over a year, despite the fact that he knew milk allergy to be one of the causes. He had learned that he could turn on the intestinal inflammation, colitis, by eating even the smallest amount of milk, cheese, or yogurt. Other food allergy symptoms dated back to childhood, when he had frequent headaches and lapses of consciousness in school. He was rejected for military service because of eczema. As an adult he still suffered with uncontrollable drowsiness and spells of anxiety and palpitations after meals, symptoms that would appear to be in part due to cerebral allergy. He fainted after being skin-tested to both milk and wheat. His bloody colitis had come upon him after a trip to Africa and was probably triggered by intestinal parasites, which would attract T-lymphocytes to the intestinal lining. The lymphocytes found milk proteins from his diet as well as the parasites, and thus local allergy developed to both. However, the parasite must have disappeared since the acute dysentery cleared up. But milk is a recurrent part of his environment.

Being a highly intelligent man, Donald had already experimented with nutrient supplements and brewer's yeast before consulting me and had already improved. However, the hair test showed low levels of manganese, iron, and zinc, and so I prescribed a supplement program with these minerals in more generous proportion. He improved remarkably, enough to actually tolerate small amounts of wheat and milk without any diarrhea. It appeared that increased zinc was particularly effective in this regard. On repeat of the hair test, six months later, all his minerals were entirely normal.

Cerebral symptoms of fatigue and drowsiness persisted until he started niacin. A 50-milligram dose produced a flush response but was not helpful. Above 400 milligrams the flush no longer occurred. Neither did his symptoms, which he rated as 95 percent reduced. He was, he said, no longer aware of them.

The orthocarbohydrate diet was also of great benefit in this case. Since the major allergens were high-carbohydrate foods, he experienced great and almost immediate relief of symptoms at the low-carbohydrate, ketosis stage early in this procedure. He no longer was in ketosis when he increased his carbohydrate intake to 50 grams per day, and he felt "exceedingly comfortable."

Since so many of my patients respond to micronutrient supplements and the orthocarbohydrate diet, I do not find it necessary to put many through a complete battery of allergy tests or the additional expense and trouble of a pulse test diet or other elimination diet. However, when the simple approach doesn't work, the more tedious and thorough method of complete allergy diagnosis and testing and treatment is essential.

Leslie is an example of a case where the orthocarbohydrate diet didn't work. A thirty-five-year-old nurse, she was quite well until she suffered an acute viral illness, possibly hepatitis, a year before consulting me. She had self-treated with vitamin A after reading a nutrition book and soon developed blurred vision and pain in her legs. The fact that she could not tolerate vitamin A supplements is further evidence of liver disease, with consequent inability to store vitamin A normally in the liver. She had also become intolerant of fats and was constipated.

When I attempted to treat her with vitamin supplements she experienced nausea and headaches. It turned out that she had always been quite allergic and suffered allergic rhinitis and eczema since childhood. Now her allergist found her allergic to "everything." She was tested by placing small amounts of substances under her tongue. After food colors and additives her heart began to race. Wheat caused her legs to tingle. Yeast made her acutely anxious, as if everything were closing in on her. Soybean made her extremely fatigued. A trial on niacin supplementation brought on a flush but also some relief of her allergy symptoms. However, the orthocarbohydrate diet made her much worse, and she terminated treatment with me. A year later she wrote to tell me of her further experience in treating her symptoms from the allergic approach. While I don't think the cause of her illness, the hepatitis, has been accounted for in her report, I am sure you will gain from her description and I agree with her conclusions.

> My problem was all allergy. I became toxic on all the vitamins and overloading of proteins on the low-carbohydrate diet. I was passing out after meals. When I started the allergy treatment I got much better. Those patients of yours who do not respond to treatment are probably allergic. The testing and treatment for ecologic illness is long and complicated but it works.

As a sidelight on this case, it happened that she told a friend about her partial benefits with niacin. I also got a letter from this friend, which I include because it documents the diversity of responses, not only to the allergy conditions, but also to the treatments. When viewed from the perspective of orthomolecular medicine, each case is an individual one.

> A year ago I got poison oak and later developed symptoms around my eyes of itching, discoloration, loss of lashes, puffiness and excessive tears. Allergy tests showed I was allergic to horses, cats, dust and certain weeds. I received temporary and inadequate relief from antihistamines; with six treatments of acupuncture I obtained partial relief, on one side.
> After eight months of this I started on 250 milligrams of niacin with meals and all symptoms disappeared. After ten days I stopped the niacin and all the symptoms returned. Thereafter and to this day I take 250 milligrams of niacin each morning with no recurrence of allergic symptoms or other side effects, including depression. I want to thank you for the cure and resumption of living with a cat, riding horses and enjoying grasses and foods.

As a doctor I am highly gratified by this woman's wonderful response to the anti-allergic effects of niacin. However, I am cautious because I have seen a few of my patients prove oversensitive to niacin and develop excessive amounts of skin irritation, hives, and in one case bowel irritation, leading to an episode of cerebral allergy with a half day of paranoid feelings, a sort of temporary schizophrenia. It is always wise to start with a small dose and build up gradually. If the flush reaction proves too uncomfortable or appears to trigger off rather than suppress allergies, niacin should not be used. On the other hand, in most cases, as the dose is increased (usually over 400 milligrams), the skin flush response, which lasts half an hour or so, will no longer occur. It is when the flush no longer occurs that the anti-allergic and anti-inflammatory benefits are most pronounced. I have been most cautious in cases of asthma, because I have observed increased wheezing with niacin supplementation at times. There is much more to be learned about how best to use this valuable nutrient. I strongly advise that you consult your own physician if you are thinking of trying niacin for yourself.

There is no doubt that nutrients have much value in our treatment of allergic disorders. There is much that we have yet to learn about their full potential. Until the advent of the new medicine of orthomolecular nutrition, our researchers and scientists did not actively study these potential benefits. They seemed too incredible! Yet the first step in taking advantage of the benefits of nutrient therapy is to believe that it is possible. Remember the case of Wendy: even though she knew she was allergic to certain foods, she couldn't bring herself to "assiduously" avoid them until she consulted an expert. My greatest value to her, I must admit, was that I helped her to believe what she already knew.

The Nutrition Prescription for Allergies

• Build up your body defenses against allergens with orthomolecular nutrition
• Hasten the removal of food allergens by increasing bowel transit time with the addition of dietary fiber and Lactobacillus acidophilus tablets or culture as well as titration (gradually increasing doses) of magnesium oxide to your requirements
• Be aware that allergy can produce cerebral symptoms as well as local tissue inflammation
• Identify allergies with the pulse test elimination diet or the three- or four-day water fast and elimination diet
• Strengthen the anti-inflammatory system by proper use of niacin, pantothenic acid, and other nutrients
• Take advantage of the hormone-sparing action of the orthocarbohydrate diet
• Remember, the low-carbohydrate diet, especially if it produces ketosis, can lower the insulin level and thus reduce allergic inflammation
• Always believe in your ability to heal

13

Vitamin C:
The Common Cure

In the annals of medicine I believe the year 1978 will go down as a turning point in the acceptance of the nutritional approach to health I am advocating in this book. In November of that year Dr. Linus Pauling addressed the annual convention of the American Medical Association. Dr. Pauling's appearance before the AMA went unnoticed in the general press, but the symbolic impact of the belated acceptance of the "Vitamin C man" by organized medicine ushered in a new era for doctors and patients alike.

To see why this is so, let me go back a few years and recount the struggles of Dr. Pauling and the followers of orthomolecular medicine to earn the respect of their colleagues. Medical progress, like any other human enterprise, isn't entirely a matter of science. It is also a matter of politics. I learned this truth the hard way when I received national publicity in *Prevention* magazine in June 1972. I was cited in an article there as a leader in the new field of nutritional therapy in psychiatry. Although I was honored by the description, I confess I wasn't aware of any such distinction at the time: all I knew was that I had accumulated my first 1,000 cases in orthomolecular work over a three-year period and seemed to be achieving valid results. Then the ax fell. A local newspaper wrote up the story and promptly a letter to the editor appeared from my local medical society, branding my views as "unscientific" and "not . . . representative of good medical practice."

At the time I was almost alone in the practice of orthomolecular medicine in Northern California. I shall never forget the support I received from an unexpected source. The shock of being branded by my peers as incompetent in my chosen field of work was overcome by the appearance of a great battler in my corner, Dr. Pauling.

Vitamin C and the Fear of Panaceas

Although Dr. Pauling's work in nutrition began as long ago as 1954—at Caltech with research on the molecular basis of mental disease—he didn't receive national attention until the publication of his award-winning *Vitamin C and the Common Cold* in 1970. The medical establishment was quick to use the press against Pauling. A flurry of newspaper stories attempted to ridicule his main contention—that large doses of C could reduce the number of common colds or mitigate their severity. With the courtesy and tact of a great teacher, however, Dr. Pauling persevered against his critics and met their skepticism with a search for more comprehensive and persuasive studies. Most of all, he wasn't afraid to put his reputation—as a humanitarian and a man of science—on the line. Yet here he was defending a most implausible proposition: there is a panacea for most of our ills, and it turns out to be a well-known vitamin!

As we will see in this chapter, the case for vitamin C as a "common cure" is overwhelming and grows every year. Yet there existed in 1970—and there still exists today—an unwillingness in medical schools as well as in physicians' offices to examine the evidence. The very idea of a cure-all is repugnant to the scientific mind. How can a single agent be effective against cancer and also against hay fever? Granted that the one-disease, one-cure theory is a thing of the past, isn't a panacea theory equally unlikely? Pauling met this obvious criticism with insights from several disciplines—chemistry, biology, anthropology. Most important to orthomolecularists like me back in 1972, this double winner of the Nobel Prize lent his prestige to the unpopular field of clinical nutrition and gave us support in research into micronutrients with far less visibility than vitamin C.

In my case, my medical society had announced that "although so-called trace elements such as magnesium are necessary for brain function, the amounts required are so minute and so prevalent in ordinary

food substances it is almost inconceivable that anybody with any semblance of a normal diet could be lacking in these trace elements." In my
practice I had taken that "inconceivable" position. Physicians who dare
to innovate must be prepared to defend their positions or face the loss
of hospital privileges or licensing. How much innovation would have
occurred in the last ten years in the field of clinical nutrition if Dr.
Pauling had not led the way with his own daring research into megavitamin therapy?

One could surmise that it was largely Dr. Pauling's maverick reputation regarding vitamin C and the common cold that led the *Proceedings
of the National Academy of Sciences* to turn down a paper in 1972.
The paper was titled "Ascorbic Acid and the Glycosominoglycans: A
Contribution to the Orthomolecular Treatment of Cancer," and its authors were Pauling and Ewan Cameron, a Scottish researcher. The NAS
had had a policy for the 58 years of its existence to publish papers of its
members. It decided to change that policy to reject a paper of member
Pauling. The editorial board of the NAS claimed the paper would "raise
false hopes" in cancer victims.

As it turned out, a magazine devoted to cancer research, *Oncology,*
accepted the paper for publication sight unseen as soon as word of the
NAS decision leaked out. Characteristically, Pauling and his colleague
were content to avoid political confrontations and let their work speak
for itself. I believe the force of their message is all the more powerful
because of that admirable scientific stance. In any case, this historic
breakthrough (*Oncology* had never before published a paper without it
being "refereed" by a panel of experts) was one of the first signals that
the Recommended Daily Allowance of a vitamin had little to do with its
potential value to health and that the whole theory of vitamins was in
for a severe shake-up.

From Forager to Farmer: Why We Have
Vitamin C Deficiency

The idea that vitamins are needed only in small doses is the unfortunate
legacy of some of the early discoveries of vitamin deficiencies. When the
Scottish physician James Lind pinpointed the cause of scurvy in 1753,
he noted that it could be prevented with a regular intake of citrus fruits.
This information was used half a century later by the British Navy:
limes were provided to Admiral Nelson's seamen, and for the first time
in history crews were able to stay at sea for longer than two or three

months. Dr. Albert Szent-Györgyi isolated the anti-scurvy agent in citrus fruit as ascorbic acid, or ascorbate, named vitamin C, in 1928, for which work he received the Nobel Prize. And Dr. William Hodges later determined that only 10 milligrams a day of ascorbate were sufficient to prevent symptoms of scurvy. When the Recommended Dietary Allowances were first laid down by the Food and Nutrition Board in 1943, Dr. Hodges' work was used as the basis for the RDA for vitamin C. Since that time, various official recommendations for daily intake of ascorbate have ranged from 30 to 60 milligrams per day, or well under one-tenth of a gram a day! No vitamin C tablet is sold today in amounts that small.

The very name "RDA" conjures up such authority, however, that a brief history of that rubric is in order. There are actually two RDAs today: the Recommended *Dietary* Allowance of the Food and Nutrition Board and the Recommended *Daily* Allowance as propagated by the Food and Drug Administration, beginning in 1973. The FDA entered the nutrition field in 1963, under the umbrella of its concern for the marketing of drugs, when it promulgated the Minimum Daily Requirements, or MDRs. That name has now all but disappeared from view, but the RDAs linger on. Scarcely a year after the FDA announced its RDAs in 1973 (based on the 1968 RDAs of the Food and Nutrition Board), the Food and Nutrition Board issued new values for *its* RDAs. Without any obvious evidence of diminishing human needs for vitamins and minerals, the standards were generally lowered. Vitamin C was reduced to 45 milligrams per day. Senator William Proxmire commented at the time:

> There is a very simple and quite unscientific reason for this. . . . The Food and Nutrition Board . . . is both the creature of the food industry and is heavily financed by the food industry. It is the narrow economic interest of the industry to establish low official RDAs because the lower the RDAs the more nutritional their food products appear.
>
> (CONGRESSIONAL RECORD, *June 10, 1974*)

The Food and Nutrition Board was established by the National Research Council of the National Academy of Sciences in 1940 and continues to be staffed by scientists who are consultants to drug or food companies or whose academic chairs are funded by them.

If the purpose of the RDAs is merely to set levels that can prevent "some terrible disease," in Proxmire's words, in the case of vitamin C the disease is practically nonexistent nowadays. The symptoms of scurvy are bleeding gums, mental depression, internal bleeding, weakened tissues, separated joints, loss of resistance to bacterial and viral infections, and eventually death from hemorrhage or infection. Except in cases of obvious malnutrition or alcoholism, scurvy isn't likely to be considered a plausible diagnosis. What, then, does Pauling mean when he suggests that an optimal intake of ascorbate is in the range of several grams a day—for him personally 10 grams? Simply this: we should be concerned not with gross manifestations of scurvy but with a sort of latent scurvy whose effects on our health are far more difficult to detect and indeed do not require medical care. Dr. Irwin Stone, a pioneer vitamin C researcher who first brought ascorbate to Pauling's attention, calls this condition "chronic subclinical scurvy" (CSS) and contends that it is present throughout the population as a contributing factor in a wide variety of other ailments. Perhaps 10 milligrams of ascorbate can prevent outright scurvy, but several grams a day are needed to overcome the effects of CSS.

It is on this critical point—that human beings have a built-in vitamin C deficiency—that Pauling's whole rationale for ascorbate as a common cure turns. He reasons, from the biochemical point of view that is his life's work, that a chemical of the complexity of ascorbate would not be synthesized *to excess* by the animals who have the ability to manufacture it in their bodies. "The dog, the cat, the rat, the mouse and other animals make their own vitamin C," he argues, and when the amount they synthesize is projected as a ratio to body weight the analogous amount appropriate to a human being ranges from a low of 3 grams a day to a high of 19. Yet the average human diet of 2500 calories a day from 110 possible plant sources yields only 2.3 grams of vitamin C a day under ideal conditions. Conclusion: human beings have a deficiency of ascorbate of from 0.7 to 16.7 grams a day.

Why some animals, *most* animals, require vitamins exogenously— from sources outside their bodies, namely food or supplements—is the key to Stone's and Pauling's explanation of man's unusual need for ascorbate. Plant life manufactures vitamins in abundance, and when animals evolved from plant life they also synthesized vitamins A, the B complex, C, and the rest. In time, however, mutants appeared who had lost the genes necessary to produce the enzymes used in making vitamins. Without this machinery, they were "streamlined" animals, as Pauling puts it, who eventually won out in the evolutionary struggle. These simpler, hardier animals got their vitamins in food. The underlying definition of a vitamin, in fact, is that it is an organic substance essential to health but not producible by the body.

In the case of ascorbate, however, many animals still manufacture enough to meet their own needs, probably because there is simply not enough available in plant food. The more clever animals, such as human beings and apes, were able to range farther afield and so shed their ascorbate-producing mechanism. Those species who were either too slow or unable to convert glucose to ascorbic acid have long since died out.

Unfortunately, another major shift in evolutionary history intervened in man's development at the dawn of civilization in the Stone Age. He began to move from the green jungle to the asphalt jungle. While ascorbate grows on trees in the form of fruits and vegetation, the trees then became harder to find. Our ancestors in the Middle Eastern Fertile Crescent gradually changed from foragers to farmers; grains and nuts, with almost no ascorbate, replaced fruits and leaves in their diet. I would say that this development ushered in what we now call medical practice. And for all this time we have been treating illness and disease without understanding their roots in our depleted diet—depleted especially of C.

Rethinking Medicine Against a Deficiency Background

In the education of a medical student, most of the studies in clinical medicine have presented the extreme cases, the "classical cases." These typically involve patients who necessarily are low in resistance to disease, for otherwise it's unlikely their cases would be so severe. But low resistance may mean nothing more than ascorbate deficiency, if Pauling's general analysis and the specific illnesses and diseases we will shortly discuss are any indication. We are therefore faced with the distinct possibility that our medical textbooks and instruction are training doctors to recognize disease only in cases of vitamin C deficiency! We may find that when all our patients are given the benefits of optimal-dose ascorbic acid, even the most feared infectious diseases, currently treated only with antibiotics, will vanish from our medical practice.

The great epidemics of infectious diseases throughout history, such as the plagues of the Middle Ages, may well have been prepared by centuries of gradual depletion of ascorbate in the diet. A dietary fad apparently began in the ninth century, when medical opinion of the time singled out fruits as unhealthful. The Medical School at Salerno, in a textbook, *Regimen Sanitatus Salernicum*, prescribed: *"Let thee have physicians three: Doctor Quiet, Doctor Merry, and Doctor Diet."* . . . followed by a *proscription* of fruits or fruit juices, on the theory that they caused dysentery. Indeed, both grape juice and wine had been conspicuously consumed by the ruling classes of the Roman Empire, and its decline and fall were accompanied by epidemics of diarrhea and mental and physical deterioration. What the ancient physicians apparently did not take into account was that the containers in which fruit juices and wine were stored were made of pewter and lined with lead. The active acids in the liquids leached lead from the lining of the containers, causing dysentery (lead colic) and deterioration of the brain and nervous system (encephalopathy). Perhaps the fall of an empire can be traced to lead poisoning.

By banning fruits and fruit juices from the everyday diet, the doctors of a millennium ago may have prevented lead poisoning in Europe, but in its place came the pox, the plague, and consumption. Wherever ascorbate-rich nutrition exists in the modern world, these diseases have declined. Of course, good sanitation and vaccines also played a role, but it's not unreasonable to assume that ascorbate deficiency was a major factor in the epidemic proportions of these diseases wherever they occurred. Even in the case of smallpox, the course of the disease depends on the resistance of the individual, a factor related to adequate ascorbate in the tissues.

The resistance to almost all disease, in the end, is correlated with vitamin C intake. To see why, we must review the evidence point by point.

Starting with the Common Cold

A chance remark by Dr. Pauling, that he would "like to live another ten or fifteen years," prompted a letter to him from Dr. Irwin Stone, who said that he would like to see him live another fifty years. This was in 1966. Stone's prescription to Pauling was a high-level ascorbate regimen, which he had been developing for 30 years. Pauling regarded the 50-year figure as unrealistic, but he took Stone's advice. After a short time he noticed a feeling of increased well-being and a striking decrease in the severity and number of colds he caught.

This was the beginning of Pauling's historic investigation of vitamin C. He was particularly intrigued by the number of early research efforts in ascorbic acid, dating back to 1934. In the postwar enthusiasm for the new antibiotics, these studies had been all but forgotten. What Pauling brought to bear on this neglected and often misinterpreted work was the power of statistical and analytical probing that had brought him to pre-eminence in the field of chemical bonding. Pauling was an early investigator of the structure of the DNA molecule, won the Nobel Prize for chemistry in 1954, and with colleagues unraveled the molecular basis of sickle-cell anemia. He now set about to fit together the pieces of the puzzle of the common cold from both epidemiological studies and laboratory research.

The anti-viral and antibacterial effects of ascorbate have been observed in the laboratory repeatedly since the 1930s. Confirming this early work, biochemists Patricia and Carlton Schwerdt recently examined a virus that produces cold symptoms and exposed it to vitamin C. The virus was severely limited in reproduction. Similarly, Dr. Claus W. Jungeblut demonstrated in 1935 that ascorbic acid inactivates the poliomyelitis virus. Other viruses have been shown to be inactivated by ascorbate in varying degrees: herpes, vaccinia, hoof and mouth, and rabies. Bacterial viruses were 99 percent inactivated by exposure for an hour to ascorbate concentrations that can be achieved in the bloodstream with large supplementary intake in studies performed by Dr. A. Murata and his coworkers in 1975. The size of ascorbate doses necessary to offer anti-viral protection is crucial and explains the contradictory results in otherwise well-managed tests.

Drs. R. Hume and E. Weyers reported in the *Scottish Medical Journal* in 1973 that on the first day of a cold the average concentration of ascorbic acid in the white blood cells (leucocytes) drops to a level of about *half* the amount sufficient to kill bacteria. To maintain an effective concentration of vitamin C in the leucocytes, one has to take a gram of ascorbate a day, and 6 grams a day for three days when a cold is contracted. A person taking ten times the RDA of vitamin C would not receive protection against bacterial infection. Dr. Murata's work at Fukuoka Hospital confirms this finding. He noted that of 150 patients receiving blood transfusions 11 contracted hepatitis. By giving successive patients at least 2 grams of ascorbate a day, he completely eliminated hepatitis cases in the next 1,100 transfusions! Now this hospital routinely prescribes from 6 to 10 grams of vitamin C a day for all its surgical and intensive-care patients—without any danger of side effects.

Dr. Stone documents the effectiveness of ascorbate against hepatitis and many other common viral diseases: fever blisters, shingles, viral pneumonia, measles, chicken pox, viral encephalitis, mumps, and infectious mononucleosis. From all of this laboratory work and clinical experience with ascorbate against infections, one could certainly make a presumptive case for vitamin C against the common cold. Numerous physicians have simply tried ascorbate in large doses at the inception of any disease or illness, and their success in one area has encouraged them to go on to the next. Two doctors in particular have expanded our clinical experience with vitamin C to all the maladies mentioned above and more: Dr. Robert Cathcart, of Incline Village, Nevada, and Dr. Frederick R. Klenner, of Reidsville, North Carolina.

As impressive as this evidence is, however, it's not the sort of scientific test that medical researchers consider conclusive. Laboratory results and clinical experience must be confirmed by controlled studies of large numbers of cases, especially if side effects are suspected. I should like to point out that one of the most attractive features of vitamin C is that it has virtually no harmful side effects. Several minerals do, of course, and vitamin D in exceptionally large doses can be fatal. But it seems to me that there's a lot of misguided fervor about testing ascorbate when hundreds of potent drugs with *known side effects* of some magnitude are accepted by the average physician. Nevertheless, large studies of vitamin C have been performed—in this case merely to determine if its effectiveness lives up to laboratory and clinical results.

Pauling's 1970 book on the common cold marshaled this evidence. The stir following its publication led to further studies, of the "double-blind" type: subjects would take either vitamin C or a placebo resembling ascorbate in taste and size, and neither group would know which pill it was taking—*and the researchers wouldn't know either.* Pauling reviewed the 13 largest studies in 1975. He found that the seven studies that were in his opinion properly carried out showed a reduction in illness of 44 percent with ascorbate and a reduction in frequency of colds of 56 percent. The remaining six studies had defects, he felt, but still showed an average protection of 19 percent against the common cold. One major study has been reported since that time (*JAMA,* March 2, 1979: "Vitamin C Prophylaxis in Marine Recruits," Henry A. Pitt, M.D., and Anthony M. Costrini, M.D.). Since this study concluded that vitamin C is of "no benefit" in preventing the common cold, a few comments should be made about Pauling's case at the moment.

Is ascorbate effective against the common cold? The "marine recruit" study is the only apparent evidence to the contrary. In reality, however, this contrary evidence tends to highlight several important points about vitamin therapy that would otherwise have been overlooked or minimized. First of all, vitamins don't operate in a vacuum, singly, or with a few nutrients. Pauling emphasizes that a deficiency in vitamin A or the B-complex vitamins can negate most of the effectiveness of ascorbate. And this study in particular involved subjects under conditions of great stress, basic training. In the eight-week study period, 90 percent of the recruits reported at least one cold. The vitamin C dose tested was 2 grams per day, and it wasn't increased at the onset of a cold. From the information reported in the *JAMA* article, we don't know anything about preexisting conditions among the subjects or their diets. All we've learned is that ascorbate in this dose and against this background appears to be no better than a placebo against the common cold. And one more thing: 8 of the 674 recruits contracted pneumonia; only 1 of those was among the ascorbate group. In a study in which so many variables were not taken into account, perhaps this is the only result worthy of mention.

Vitamin C against Cholesterol

Few people die of the common cold, but heart disease is another matter. Why then has there been so much publicity over vitamin C and the common cold when ascorbate has shown surprising results against the major risk factors in atherosclerosis? The evidence is there for anyone to see, and Pauling called attention to it at the same time as he began to publish the evidence for ascorbate against the common cold.

As we have seen, "cholesterol" has become a scare word and its significance is often misunderstood. We must carefully distinguish between (1) dietary cholesterol and blood cholesterol; (2) blood cholesterol and cholesterol deposits in damaged walls of arteries; and (3) the favorable and unfavorable types of carriers of cholesterol, HDL and LDL. None of the three is necessarily related. Yet ascorbate seems to play a role in reducing the damaging aspects of cholesterol in all three cases.

• The higher the vitamin C concentration, the lower the cholesterol in the blood and liver. Dr. Emil Ginter reported in 1973 that a study of guinea pigs showed ascorbate is essential for the conversion of cholesterol into acids excreted in the bile. A level of ascorbate intake comparable to that of the RDA for human beings did not efficiently remove excess cholesterol from the body by way of bile acids. More is required.

• The lack of vitamin C is correlated with damaged blood vessels. Dr. G. C. Willis found that atherosclerosis in guinea pigs was reversed by sufficiently high intakes of ascorbate; in some cases damaged blood vessels were completely healed. Willis also studied human aortas at autopsy and found that the lowest amounts of vitamin C measurable in the vessels were correlated with the worst damage to the vessels.

• The higher the vitamin C, the higher the HDL cholesterol. In 1977 Dr. C. J. Bates and associates reported in *Lancet* that high-density lipoprotein, which helps transport cholesterol out of tissues, is associated with the presence of high levels of ascorbate.

In the light of these promising indications it is astounding that research dollars continue to pour into other aspects of heart disease while very little attention is paid to vitamin C or other vitamin therapy against the effects of cholesterol. On this count alone, the Framingham study is probably defective: none of the subjects in that massive test were asked about their intake of ascorbate or of foods rich in vitamin C.

Why should vitamin C have beneficial effects against heart disease? The rationale for the action of ascorbate was first suggested by Dr. Constance Spittle, an English pathologist. She observed a drop in her serum cholesterol from 240 milligrams per deciliter to 160 after only one month of a vegetarian diet she began in 1970. As a test, she resumed her previous diet and was surprised to find the cholesterol continuing to fall. Apparently whatever was causing the cholesterol to drop could not be explained by the *absence* of something, such as animal fat, but by the presence of a nutrient. Dr. Spittle observed that even a high-cholesterol diet was accompanied by a drop in serum cholesterol when the diet included a large amount of fresh fruit and vegetables. Further, cooking the vegetables, which destroys vitamin C, led to an increase in serum cholesterol. She decided to test the implication that ascorbate was responsible for controlling serum cholesterol, and in the process uncovered a clue to the way the vitamin works in the human body.

Fifty-eight volunteers were given a gram of vitamin C a day for six weeks and were checked periodically for cholesterol levels. Among the group were 25 atherosclerotic patients. Surprisingly, this group showed a rise in blood cholesterol, as did the older subjects in general. In the younger subjects, cholesterol levels fell. Dr. Spittle reasoned that ascorbate must in some way mobilize deposits of cholesterol from the arterial walls faster than the body can get rid of it. She reasoned that treatment should involve continuing vitamin C therapy until the blood cholesterol level would come down and it did. Her general conclusion that atherosclerosis is an ascorbate-deficiency disease has more logic to it than the continuing barrage of warnings about the dangers of animal fat in the diet.

It's natural enough to look at a vegetarian diet from the point of view of what it omits rather than what it contains. In his syndicated newspaper column "Keeping Fit," Dr. Lawrence Power recently wrote:

> A colleague of mine died for a few minutes several years ago. He stopped breathing and had no pulse during a heart attack, but was brought back to life by modern help. One miracle is all he expects in his lifetime, so now he watches the food he eats. . . . He went through the corn oil phase . . . yet his blood cholesterol levels hung steadily at 230, still very much in heart attack country. Then my colleague learned that the average vegetarian's cholesterol was 150, so he quit meat for six weeks and watched his own levels slip below 200. . . . He persuaded several patients with chest pain from heart disease to stop eating all animal products. They did and within 6 months were completely relieved of their symptoms. . . . My colleague who turned to a meat-free solution for his coronary artery disease is convinced that vegetarianism is the answer.

I wonder if the meat-free solution isn't really a vitamin C-rich solution in disguise.

Vitamin C versus the "Big C"

No one dares predict what Linus Pauling will turn his attention to next, but if he had done nothing before his work on cancer and nothing after, his reputation would still be secure in medical history. Collaborating with Dr. Ewan Cameron, Pauling has assembled incontrovertible evidence that megadoses of ascorbate are effective against "hopeless" cases of cancer of many types. They write, "It is our opinion that supplemental ascorbate will soon attain an established place in the routine management of all forms of human cancer."

Pauling would be the first to remind us that his contribution to the subject is not one of original research but of synthesis of the work of hundreds of others over the last 40 years. Again, only a scientist of Pauling's stature could have made an impact against the ingrained prejudices of the heavily funded "cancer establishment," and the sensationalism of the common-cold controversy was perhaps a necessary preliminary for his obtaining a hearing in the general press.

As long ago as 1937, German researchers reported that patients with advanced cancer had low body concentrations of ascorbate. From 1948 to 1956 a large-scale study was made of the population of San Mateo County, in California, comparing the mortality of those who took more than the RDA of vitamin C with those who took less. Those who took more ascorbate showed a 60 percent decrease in age-corrected mortality from cancer and cardiovascular disease. These indications and dozens more, as persuasive as they are, were scarcely noticed in the medical literature until Pauling began to marshal them with the sort of clinical trials conducted by Cameron.

Why should ascorbate prove to be efficacious against cancer when billions of dollars spent on a wide range of medical theories have turned up little except more potent chemicals, surgery, and radiation? Pauling argues that ascorbate potentiates the various natural protective mechanisms of the body. In the host's resistance to cancer, a half-dozen or more factors are involved, from the immune system to the strengthening of cells. Vitamin C is necessary for them all. In our present state of evolution, we are ascorbate-deficient animals, he again reminds us. Although Pauling has only sketched the possible biochemical functioning of vitamin C against cancer cells, his general argument and his clinical evidence are difficult to ignore.

Most recently, Cameron and Pauling reported on the survival time of 100 cancer patients who agreed to take massive supplemental doses of ascorbate; all forms of conventional treatment had been stopped both for them and a control group, all "hopeless cases." The survival time of those on vitamin C was extended *more than 50 times* that of those who received no treatment. In summary he says, "The most basic argument for its use rests on the finding that cancer patients are almost invariably quite severely depleted of ascorbate."

Several recent studies have suggested the protective mechanism vitamin C may have against cancer. Dr. Robert Yonemoto notes that lymphocytes, tissue cells that are part of the body's immune system, are increased significantly with an intake of 5 grams of ascorbate a day and even more with 10 grams. Lymphocyte activity is known to correlate well with a favorable prognosis in cancer patients. Dr. Benjamin Siegel of the University of Oregon Health Sciences Center traces the effect of ascorbate through the action of several types of cells. Key elements in the body's defenses known as T-cells become sensitized by allergy or infection and release lymphokines, a sort of messenger cell, to activate anti-infecting agents. Among these are macrophages, "angry" cells that can contain and destroy virus and cancer cells. Siegel suggests that these cells are in turn enhanced by an agent known as interferon, discussed in Chapter 4. And many researchers have concluded that vitamin C stimulates the body's production of interferon as well as activates T-cells.

Headaches, Drugs, Intelligence, Snakebite, Old Age . . .

Although the name Dr. Szent-Györgyi coined for vitamin C, ascorbic acid, simply means "without scurvy," this molecule is a more versatile substance than he imagined. Quite recently, after more than 50 years since his discovery of the vitamin, he has found that ascorbate catalyzes the removal of electrons from protein. The protein thereby becomes a conductor of electricity and able to participate in the chemistry of life. It is here, at the submolecular level, that he and others expect to find the ultimate explanation for the action of vitamin C. "Life is absolutely below that level," he theorizes, "in the electronic dimension."

Two well-known functions of ascorbate seem to account for the improbable but demonstrated efficacy of the vitamin against problems as apparently unrelated as headaches and snakebite. First, ascorbate contributes to the collagen protein, the glue that holds cells together to form tissue, organs, and the overall structure of the body. Second, ascorbate is a sort of stabilizer in the thousands of chemical reactions that occur throughout the body.

If the action of ascorbate is so fundamental to the body, one would expect it to contribute to the general improvement of one's physiological age. Several epidemiological studies support this indication. Drs. Harold Chope and Lester Breslow followed 577 people over the age of fifty for seven years to study 25 health factors, one of which was the intake of vitamin C. Those who had taken as little as 125 milligrams of supplemental ascorbate a day—one-eighth of a gram—had a death rate 60 percent less than those receiving less than 25 milligrams a day. They concluded that vitamin C intake was the most important of the 25 health factors studied. In a similar study of more than a thousand physicians, dentists, and their spouses, Dr. Emanuel Cheraskin found that the number of symptoms of illness decreased as their vitamin C intake increased. Reviewing this material, Dr. Pauling estimated that an intake of 2 grams or more a day of ascorbate is associated with a physiological age of about 16 years less than those taking less than 1 gram a day.

Here are some more specific examples of ascorbate's versatility:

• Intelligence: Drs. A. L. Kubala and M. M. Katz reported a significant drop in intelligence test scores in school children taking less than 1 gram of vitamin C a day, compared with children taking a gram a day or more.

• Migraine headaches: Drs. L. Bali and E. Callaway, of the University of California Medical Center in San Francisco, reported the case of a patient who was able to clear up migraine headaches for the first time in six years by taking 6 grams of vitamin C a day. When he stopped taking the vitamin, his headaches returned. With the patient's permission, ascorbate and a placebo were given him in an irregular pattern not known to the patient or the doctors; without fail, severe headaches occurred only on the placebo days.

• Metal poisoning: several reports have been made of the beneficial effect of ascorbate against lead, mercury, and cadmium poisoning.

• Snakebite, bacterial toxins, burns: Dr. Frederick R. Klenner, of Reidsville, North Carolina, has been a pioneer in expanding the clinical application of ascorbate against a wide variety of bacterial and viral diseases, including snakebite. He uses it as a 3 percent spray to relieve pain and forestall infection in burns. He is justifiably proud of applying the little-known laboratory knowledge about vitamin C at a time when other physicians derided his description of it as a "miracle substance."

My own experience with vitamin C indeed confirms Dr. Klenner's enthusiasm. I have used ascorbate crystals in solution for local application to herpes "cold sores," both in the mouth and genitalia. Results have been practically 100 percent effective. The solution, a gram of ascorbate dissolved in ¼ cup of water, should be applied for about a minute with a cotton swab, and the application should be terminated when a burning sensation appears.

One of my patients, a forty-five-year-old woman, came to me in desperation after being told by several well-qualified physicians that the ulcers on her swollen tongue and cheeks would persist for at least six weeks. I placed her on a program of nutrient supplementation appropriate for illness (higher than usual amounts of vitamins A, E, the B complex, and minerals, especially zinc and magnesium), and swabbed the sores with the vitamin C solution. She was better in a day and had a dramatic recovery on the third day. In less severe cases I have seen cold sores cured overnight.

I have also had good results with migraine headaches and in helping patients withdraw from pain pills to which they had become addicted. Ascorbate in doses of 1 to 2 grams per hour during the acute withdrawal period offers great relief to patients withdrawing from narcotic drugs as well—codeine, Dilaudid, and heroin. Along with a program of micronutrient supplements, vitamin C definitely reduces symptoms of distress and muscle pain.

Drug rehabilitation of hard-core narcotics addicts is surely one of the most sensational accomplishments of vitamin C therapy. This modality was first researched by Drs. Irwin Stone and Albert Libby, yet this major breakthrough in the treatment of addiction has received scant attention in the general press. Many of their patients reported that the feeling of well-being was largely responsible for their ability to get off drugs comfortably and permanently: the natural high of good health replaced the drug high. Further studies reported in 1979, including one conducted at the San Francisco Drug Treatment Center, have confirmed their work.

Dr. Cathcart and the 100-Gram Cold

How is one to know how much ascorbate his or her individual body needs? The answer is surprisingly simple: what Dr. Robert Cathcart, of Incline Village, Nevada, calls "bowel tolerance." You can increase your intake of ascorbate until symptoms of diarrhea appear—and they won't appear until your system receives the amount of the vitamin it needs to counteract its illness. Under conditions of stress or infection, it has been observed that mammals who produce vitamin C in their bodies make as much as ten times more than they produce when well. If a similar ratio holds for human beings, a person who experiences diarrhea at 10 grams a day could tolerate up to 100 grams when severely ill.

Naturally, at such a high dose one should be under a doctor's care, even though the safety of ascorbate is well established. Cathcart points out that the corollary of this observation of the body's tolerance of vitamin C is that the more you can tolerate, the more you need. "If you have a 100-gram cold, and you're taking roughly 100 grams a day, you will quickly eliminate perhaps 90 percent of the symptoms of the disease. But if you treat the same cold with 2 grams or even 20 grams a day, you won't see much happen." Recall the marine recruit study reported in this chapter: even those with colds took only 2 grams a day.

Dr. Cathcart has treated more than 9,000 patients with megadoses of ascorbic acid for such diseases as influenza, viral pneumonia, mononucleosis, mumps, rubella, measles, chicken pox, and hepatitis. He has not had to hospitalize a single patient due to an infectious disease. "The important thing with mono or other responsive diseases," he says, "is that we can get people back to work in days. The other disease that is very specific is infectious hepatitis. It's a cinch for vitamin C."

The important thing to remember is that massive doses should be taken at the first signs of an illness. There *are* such things as 100-gram colds. Ten or more grams can be taken at three-hour intervals. Younger people seem to be able to tolerate the occasional discomfort of gas pains or diarrhea, especially when they see immediate results in relieving their symptoms of illness. When one feels well, a daily dose of about 4 grams is quite comfortable for most people, but one can experiment with higher doses until bowel tolerance is reached.

There are many things short of outright illness that can deplete the body's vitamin C. How much do you get in your diet? Three of the best food sources of vitamin C—an orange, a glass of cranberry juice, a serving of broccoli—each offer only about $\frac{1}{10}$ of a gram of ascorbate. Pollutants in the air, aspirin, and a number of other medications cause a substantial drain on your vitamin C reserves. There is now evidence that oral contraceptives deplete the vitamin, perhaps by increasing the rate of its breakdown. The worst vitamin C thief is cigarette smoking. A survey of 2,000 Canadians by Dr. Omer Peletier in 1975 showed that one-pack-a-day smokers lost 25 percent of their ascorbate and heavier smokers lost more than 40 percent.

It's ironic that the megadoses of vitamin C for which Pauling's work is still considered suspect by the medical establishment were the first clue in his investigation of ascorbate. He was intrigued by the reports of Drs. Abram Hoffer and Humphry Osmond, working in Canada, of their success in treating schizophrenic patients with large doses of B vitamins. Then he came across a study by Dr. H. Van der Kamp showing that chronic schizophrenic patients required 40 grams of vitamin C a day before they eliminated even a small amount in their urine. Normally one would expect vitamin C to appear in the urine at doses 100 times less. Finally, Dr. Stone brought his research on ascorbate to Pauling's attention, as we have seen, and the rest is history.

So, in an indirect way, vitamin C has also been responsible for the establishment of the Orthomolecular Medical Society, of which I am currently president. Without Pauling's interest in and popularization of ascorbate, the nutritional medicine my colleagues and I practice might still be thought to be some obscure form of quackery. And doctors who prescribe nutrition might still be taken to task by their medical society because "it is inconceivable that anybody with any semblance of a normal diet could be lacking . . ."

The Nutrition Prescription of Vitamin C

• Learn your tolerance to ascorbate by gradually increasing your daily intake (2 to 4 grams should be easily tolerated)
• Increase your intake of ascorbate drastically at the first sign of a cold or other illness, to the point of bowel intolerance
• Don't attempt to get enough vitamin C—unlike the other nutrients—from foods alone
• Take vitamin C in pills in addition to that in a multivitamin supplement
• In serious illness, such as heart disease and cancer, ask your doctor about the possibility of vitamin C treatment as a complement to traditional therapy

14

Megavitamins:
Treating the Causes
Instead of the Symptoms

The body is capable of relatively few basic reactions, but these may result from widely varying causes. How much do we really know about causes, and how much do we know about what is needed to treat them?

Prior to 1960, the concept of megadoses of vitamins was scarcely considered. Nowadays we use a hundred or a thousand times what was thought to be sufficient then. Linus Pauling has given us the rationale for such doses, not in terms of overkill, but of a principle of chemistry: the greater the concentration of molecules in a chemical reaction, the *faster* the reaction will proceed. It is the speed of chemical reactions of certain vitamin-dependent functions that has allowed us to treat the causes that we could never get at before.

The use of vitamin C against the common cold and cancer are good examples, but megadoses were first used in mental illness. Hereditary disorders of many kinds can be cured only by megadoses. Schizophrenia may be one of them. But while these disorders are rare, it is not rare at all for "normal" individuals to differ in size, shape, metabolism, and other physical endowments that are the basis of what biochemist Dr. Roger Williams has called "*biochemical individuality*." If one person needs so much of vitamin such-and-such for optimal health, another may require twice, three times, or even ten times the amount to reach the same level of health.

In the past 25 years the use of large doses of vitamins and minerals has proved useful in various mental illnesses as well as in a number of bodily disorders. The effect of niacinamide on arthritis, vitamin C on virus infections, vitamin E on leg cramps, and vitamin D on calcium disorders are just a few examples. We have also seen how selenium has proved effective in some cancer cases and silicon has been found to be beneficial in preventing CHD.

Megavitamins should be taken under the watchful eye of an experienced orthomolecular physician. Large doses of vitamins can initiate unexpected chemical reactions and these reactions can deplete other nutrients. For example, large doses of either B_{12} or folic acid seem to promote reactions that use up the other. Or when B_6 is provided in large amounts, niacin and magnesium may be depleted.

Megavitamins Do the Talking

The potential efficacy of megavitamin therapy was impressed on me by a psychiatric case in which all conventional therapies had failed. Theresa D. was preoccupied and distracted by constant auditory hallucinations. The voices of her five previous husbands had been criticizing and heckling her for years. Her sixth husband was understandably distraught with her disability; he threatened to divorce her and to retain custody of their four-year-old child. Theresa was willing to try anything: she cooperated in hypnosis therapy but the benefits were transient. The voices would leave for a few hours only to return again. She had been taking a well-known antipsychotic drug, with no effect on her hallucinations. At this point I recommended, on the strength of some promising indications in the literature, mainly Hoffer and Osmond, that she take a large dose of niacinamide. Her situation was desperate: if she did not improve promptly, she would probably have to return to the hospital for the fourth time in as many years. As vitamin therapy is relatively non-toxic, there was nothing to lose and much to be gained.

I was astounded by the results. Where "talk therapy," hypnosis, and drug therapy had been unsuccessful for several years, megavitamins made a dramatic breakthrough; in three days the voices began to subside and in a week the hallucinations were gone. Not many patients respond to niacinamide therapy this quickly, but even one case like this was persuasive. After this demonstration I would never doubt the value of megavitamins. This is not to say that megavitamins are the answer to every—or even *most*—desperate situations.

Maxine J. consulted me because of prolonged state of depersonalization: she described it as a total absence of feelings, a feeling of living death. Because she had been a psychiatric technician, she had read a book about megavitamin therapy and when she came to me was already taking large doses of niacinamide, vitamin C, vitamin E, and a multivitamin tablet. The megadoses were 2,000 milligrams of C and niacinamide three times a day. She had been taking three times as much a month earlier but had to cut down the dosage because of stomach upset. But the vitamins had no noticeable effect.

A survey of her dietary habits suggested a possible reason why not. Her *one* meal a day consisted of a hamburger, french fries, a meager bit of lettuce and tomato, and lots of coffee. Every day she drank between 25 and 30 cups! She smoked more than two packs of cigarettes a day with coffee. The reliance on vitamins in the face of this deplorable nutritional regimen was destined to fail.

It was not surprising to find that she was also susceptible to organic illness. Two years earlier she had been diagnosed as suffering from a form of allergy of the blood vessels called "Behçet's disease." This required treatment with cortisone to suppress blisters in her mouth, vagina, and eyes. Cortisone, however, aggravated her mental condition and she was hospitalized. Her loss of feelings persisted.

Where tranquilizers and megavitamins had both failed her, diet therapy now led to a return of feelings in a couple of weeks and a complete recovery in a few months. Simply adding a variety of vegetables, fruits, and nuts to her diet, and restricting her intake of coffee, did the trick. At one time she had been told that she might die from Behçet's disease within two years. Now her physical condition improved so remarkably that for the last year I saw her she did not require any cortisone. In this case, nutritional therapy was the answer, not megavitamin therapy. Even when diet is adequate megavitamins work more effectively in some illnesses—schizophrenia, for example—than others. The acute type is like a delirium or living nightmare. In chronic cases the whole personality is changed: delusions, or "crazy" ideas, are prominent. Schizophrenics hang on to their unreasonable delusions because in some way they are rewarding. Schizophrenics also suffer from an inability to compromise their beliefs in discussion with others. This is an important cause of alienation and loneliness. Unfortunately, this symptom is not likely to respond to orthomolecular treatment in chronic cases where unreasonableness has become a habit. On the other hand, even a chronic grouch is likely to improve in mood when physical well-being improves; and this can open the door to psychotherapy and the benefits of positive suggestion. Let me be emphatic about this: nutrient therapy is also a form of psychotherapy, and it facilitates other forms of psychotherapy.

Food for Thought

Dr. Carl Pfeiffer was the first, in the 1960s, to study the role of histamine for its effect on mood in schizophrenia. (A histamine is a hormone substance that causes blood vessels to dilate, i.e., it sensitizes white blood cells, leukocytes, to identify foreign bodies readily and attack them.) Patients high in histamines tend to be depressed and obsessive, while low-histamine patients tend to be overactive and suspicious. Dr. Carl Pfeiffer's work indicates that 20 percent of schizophrenics are high and 50 percent low in histamine, and another 30 percent are in a different category: "pyrroluric." Due to genetic enzyme deficiency, their body chemistry produces an excess of pyrrole molecules, which help manufacture blood pigment. While pyrrole is normally used by the body as a part of the hemoglobin molecule, if it is unused the pyrrole fragments accumulate in the blood or tissues and illness results. In the skin, excess pyrroles cause severe rashes when exposed to sunlight. In the brain and nervous system, a diversity of unpleasant symptoms can occur: headache, irritability, muscle twitching, abdominal pain, severe agitation, and acute psychosis.

Not until we knew for sure how all the things we see as functions of the mind are related to the brain and the nervous system could we begin to be scientific about mental disorders. We now consider one type of former "mental illness" a learning disorder, which accounts for states of seemingly unwarranted anxiety or antisocial behavior. Another type of mental disorder may be due to physical or chemical damage to the nervous system. Head injuries, infection of the brain, tumors, strokes, poisonings, and central nervous system diseases all lead to personality changes and disorders of feelings and thought processes. But the most common source of altered mental activity is *altered brain chemistry,* and this is associated with nutritional and metabolic conditions such as nutrient deficiency and hormonal imbalance.

Some of us are more vulnerable than others to deficiencies and imbalances because of genetics. For instance, it is known that some two dozen inborn errors of metabolism are a result of inherited enzyme deficiencies. In such cases, a vital molecule is lacking in quantity or potency so that the chemistry of life is weakened. In severe cases the individual so afflicted cannot live. In less severe cases life goes on but is severely handicapped by a malfunction of the nervous system.

These recent discoveries, which have been well documented both in research laboratories and in clinical work, are among the most exciting developments in orthomedicine. For the first time we have convincing evidence that the concentrations of foods and the nutrients they contain have a major influence on the quality of our mental responses. Heretofore, it was believed that our bodies took whatever we offered in the way of food and converted it, through digestive and hormonal action, into the proper mix of molecules for our individual needs. Now that view is not merely challenged: *it is obsolete.*

Not too long ago, it was believed that vitamin therapy was useful only in treating well-defined deficiency diseases, such as pellagra (which can produce mental illness seemingly identical to schizophrenia). Too few doctors realize that even when blood tests are normal it's possible to have a deficiency because of the effects of enzymes and tissues unrelated to blood values. For the past three-quarters of a century the psychodynamic approach—"talk therapy"—has dominated the field, and doctors haven't looked for deficiencies. Few would know what test to order to find these deficiencies. How do we explain the many cases that respond to megavitamins without the well-known clinical signs of pellagra, dermatitis, or diarrhea? And how many of these disorders were once thought to be mental disorders?

A Mental Block against Megadoses

There were 10,000 cases of pellagra treated as schizophrenia in hospitals in the South in the year 1910. However, since the work of Drs. Joseph Goldberger and Tom Spies, demonstrating the cure of pellagra with low doses of vitamin B_3, niacin, or niacin-rich foods, such as brewer's yeast, liver, or milk, it is nowadays unlikely to find even a few cases of pellagra psychosis left in our mental hospitals anywhere in this country; but there is still plenty of schizophrenia. Among our present cases there are many that could be helped by administering megadoses of niacin. We know this because thousands of patients have been helped by orthomolecular physicians since the pioneering work of Hoffer, Osmond, and Smythies in 1952.

But, even before that, there was good evidence for the use of megadose niacin therapy in treating atypical psychotic states. In plainer terms, these cases were mostly forms of schizophrenia. In 1939, Dr. Harvey Cleckley and his colleagues described a series of cases that responded dramatically to megadose niacin therapy. Patients were relieved of manic excitement, delusions, and hallucinations despite the fact that pellagra was not diagnosed and there was no clear indication for niacin treatment.

I am sure it took as much courage as wisdom for the doctors to proceed with their innovative treatment; but the results were spectacular. One patient who showed no improvement with 600 milligrams per day of niacin by mouth was cured within a matter of minutes after an intravenous injection of 800 milligrams. Another patient failed to improve on 600 milligrams of niacin per day but recovered when the dose was increased to 1500 milligrams per day.

Both patients regained their sanity in what could only be described as a miraculous fashion. Here we have the beginnings of "megavitamin therapy," with doses 100 times larger than usual in treatment of mental disorders.

The word "therapy" can also be used to identify treatment of non-mental disorders. The distinction between physical and mental has, in fact, been shown to be artificial in many instances of orthomolecular treatment. This is an essential point of orthomolecular work.

Somehow these exciting findings were brushed aside for the next ten years. Then Abram Hoffer and Humphry Osmond investigated the possibility that large doses of niacin might prevent the formation of hallucinogenic substances in the brain of schizophrenics. The psychiatric profession was still looking for answers in Freud, Jung, and other schools of psychodynamic theory; a few pharmacological pioneers were bringing in the then revolutionary tranquilizers, chemicals whose actions in the body were not well understood. But Hoffer and Osmond, along with their colleague John Smythies, were focusing on the molecular chemistry of the brain.

Their early results were so positive that they pursued their theory despite a storm of controversy. Their very first case was a dramatic success: a young man who was in danger of imminent death due to exhaustion from prolonged and uncontrollable excitement. Because he was unable to cooperate, niacin was administered by stomach tube in doses of 5 grams. In a matter of hours he was well!

There was no doubt in this case about the diagnosis. This was schizophrenia, not pellagra. It was not a simple case of vitamin deficiency, as had been claimed by some who had challenged the observations of Cleckley, Sydenstricker, and Geeslin.

For almost ten years Hoffer and Osmond worked to establish the ground rules to make this form of treatment available. They ran some of the most refined clinical trials in psychiatry to prove their theory. Their initial report, issued in 1957, indicated 17 out of 21 patients (83 percent) recovered on niacin treatment, compared with 3 out of 9 recoveries (33 percent) in a control group of schizophrenics not treated with vitamins. In a larger study of patients followed for nine years, Hoffer and Osmond found that only 10 percent of 73 schizophrenics treated with megadoses of vitamins remained in the hospital and there were no suicides. Of 98 patients not treated with vitamins, half remained in the hospital and there were 4 suicides.

Finally, in 1962, Hoffer persuaded a group of physicians who were not enthusiastic about vitamin therapy to administer megadoses of niacin to 128 patients. These patients accumulated 7,422 days in the hospital among them during the study. This time was dramatically less than the 54,491 days in the hospital accumulated by a similar comparison group who were not given niacin.

Further research soon revealed that vitamin therapy worked quite well in those patients who had been ill only a short time. Results in chronic patients, however, whose personalities had deteriorated due to illness and the loss of normal life experiences, are not impressive. Still, even in chronic cases *some* benefits were observed by Patrick O'Reilly, who studied eleven of "the most refractory, regressed, and deteriorated female patients" at the Saskatchewan Hospital. Although he claimed no success in curing their diseases with megadose niacin, he rated them— after an average of 16 years in the hospital—as improved after just 8 weeks on niacin in the following areas:

- Sleep improved in all patients.
- Appetite increased in all.
- Directability improved in six.
- Initiative better in five.
- Cooperation in hospital routine better in four.
- Care of personal property improved in three.

This result compared with the fact that patients in a similar group not treated with megadoses of niacin showed no improvement at all.

Which Therapy Is in the Patient's Interest?

Why there should be such resistance to megadose and mega-nutrition therapy among so many intelligent physicians and administrators is hard to explain. It seems unreasonable that vitamin and mineral therapy is shunned and sometimes forbidden in our healing institutions while our well-accepted pharmacological drug therapies are *known* to be toxic. It's especially puzzling when there seems to be unanimous agreement among those who have looked into megavitamin therapy for schizophrenia that it does work, sometimes dramatically. Nevertheless, it's a fact that the attitude of the medical and the nursing professions toward this therapy has been negative. Hospitals have been unwilling to allow patients to be treated with vitamin therapy—not only megadose therapy, but even the inclusion of complete vitamin supplements and the avoidance of excesses of sugar and coffee.

Two double-blind studies showed a 50 percent reduction in the time of recovery for hospitalized acute schizophrenics with the simple expedient of removing wheat and milk from their diet! Yet, somehow this simple dietary change is a message that hasn't reached most of our hospitals and the physicians in charge, despite the fact that successful reports were published over ten years ago in a 1968 study by Dr. Francis Dohan, which showed wheat to cause irritability and paranoia.

I have known some doctors who have been ostracized by their professional colleagues over the question of megadose therapy. Certified psychiatrists have been accused of incompetence when they claimed results were positive with this type of treatment. I have personally treated two registered nurses whose health and careers were saved by megadose niacin and orthomolecular treatment; yet both felt they had to keep this fact secret lest they be fired from their jobs.

One of these nurses was a thirty-five-year-old I'll call Laura. She was unmarried, dependent upon her job for a livelihood. When she became depressed over an extended period, she discovered that taking 100 milligrams of niacin every few hours kept her cheerful, mentally alert, and free from the anxious self-consciousness that she'd had all her life. She credited the vitamin with saving her job and perhaps her life. While she was relieved to find in me a doctor to whom she could talk about it freely, she nevertheless was terribly afraid that someone at work would find out she took such high doses of niacin and that it would cost her

her job. It was the attitude of her colleagues that vitamin therapy is quackery.

I personally became involved in orthomolecular treatment because, while I was reasonably satisfied with the results of psychotherapy for my "healthy" patients, I was disappointed in it in the more difficult cases of schizophrenia, chronic depression, alcoholism, and drug addiction. My results indicated that 80 to 90 percent of my patients suffering from anxiety, phobia, and acute depression were cured or much improved with hypnosis and behavioral therapy methods. Those with schizophrenia, chronic depression and addictions suffered relapses in two-thirds of the cases. I began investigating dietary patterns in depth and I was astounded to find that the dietary habits of many of my patients were inadequate. It was so obvious: here was an untapped source of healing power whose indications were strongly supported by objective data from the laboratory studies of vitamin and mineral levels in blood and hair.

Because of the prevalence of undernutrition among my patients, I made it a point to hold off megadose treatment until the possible benefits of general nutritional support and nutrient supplements were tried. When I attended my first meeting of the Academy of Orthomolecular Psychiatry in 1971, a year after it was formed, I was surprised to find that this method that seemed so sensible to me was not the standard with my colleagues. It turned out that I was the only one in the group who was already using a standard nutritional history questionnaire to ducument the food intake of my patients.

I was also more dedicated to keeping all the vitamins and minerals in balance. This is not so important now that our available vitamin supplements are better balanced and more complete, but in the 1960s most of the commercially available products were neither complete nor well balanced. In particular, vitamin B_6 was often underrepresented, being present in microgram amounts rather than milligrams. Also, trace minerals were not yet appreciated, hence magnesium, zinc, manganese, and chromium were often missing from the supplements or represented in insignificant amounts. Fortunately, this situation was improved when the RDA values issued by the National Research Council were made more complete in 1974 and the manufacturers had to follow suit in order to call their products "complete."

Another factor that helped formulate my theories was a meeting with the biochemist John J. Miller. The Miller Pharmacal Company generously offered the most stimulating seminars in nutritional medicine available at that time, and I learned from them that adequacy of trace minerals made the use of megadose vitamins unnecessary in many cases. This certainly influenced me to think about the biochemical factors, pathways, and interactions rather than prescribing shotgun megadoses of everything in sight.

The "Ortho" Approach: Testing and Regulating

By adopting the name "orthomolecular," we also adopt a certain philosophy, one in which the importance of *all* the nutrients is appreciated. What once was exclusive to a few megavitamins is now a more complete, total nutritional approach. Thus, it is now usual to survey the diet by means of computer analysis to analyze the blood chemistries, including water- and fat-soluble vitamins, and to document the nutrient state of the tissues. We also study the mineral levels in blood, urine, and hair. Hair analysis of minerals is used not only for diagnostic purposes, but also to monitor the nutritional state of the patient until treatment benefits are achieved and the effects of the program have been stabilized.

As a pioneer in developing this method of diet and hair analysis, my path took me away from megavitamin treatment to such an extent that I was worried I might be missing something my colleagues were seeing. It was unusual for my patients to take more than 3 grams of niacin or niacinamide a day; yet other doctors were prescribing 20 grams per day or more. There were many reports of patients who did not respond until more than 12 grams per day were given. And I can attest to one particularly excitable young man who had gone on a rampage and didn't calm down until he took 40 grams of niacin a day. I also recall a number of patients who were benefited by niacin or niacinamide treatment but who stopped taking the vitamins through carelessness or complacency and then suffered a relapse. These cases seemed to have a demoralizing effect on the patients and it proved difficult to regain the advantages once enjoyed with niacin therapy. Was it a good idea to overprescribe to hedge one's bets? I became convinced that the challenge of the orthomolecular approach was to provide the *optimal,* "ortho" amount of vital nutrients. The difference between megadose and optimal dose is occasionally the difference between harmful side effects and no side effects. My instincts have always been to keep vitamin doses at the lowest level that will get the job done and to back off whenever there is a suspicion of bad effects from large vitamin doses. As a rule, if adverse reactions occur, I advise my patients to reduce the dose of vitamins or minerals or discontinue them until we have a chance to review their responses.

In practice, then, the method of gradually increasing the dose, observing the results, and increasing the dose some more is the best way to determine the optimal dose. There is no other test that is as accurate as the total response of the patient to vitamin therapy. For example, it is possible to provide 50 to 100 milligrams of B vitamins in a single tablet. With this as a starting point it is a simple matter to gradually increase the two B vitamins most likely to be helpful at large doses: B_3 (niacin) and B_6 (pyridoxine). These are increased 100 milligrams per dose, three times per day, until benefits are noted or until nausea, stomach upset, or headache indicate the patient has surpassed his or her individual tolerance level. Niacinamide is often preferred over niacin because it does not cause the marked skin flush; however, the results are not always interchangeable. There are some who respond better to niacin.

As a rule I recommend that, where megadoses are considered likely to provide a possible benefit, patients start with niacinamide and then add a small dose of niacin. The dose is increased gradually until a distinct flush reaction of the skin occurs within an hour or two. At this point, a stimulating effect is often noted. Some of my patients report that their mood improves and, in particular, depressed feelings are relieved. This treatment seems especially valuable in cases of mental confusion and emotional agitation, because these symptoms are often improved with higher doses of niacin. Megadose niacin has a definite tranquilizing effect for many people, especially those who suffer from schizophrenic symptoms. In fact, results with niacin are often better than from the use of chemical tranquilizers because the mind remains clearer. However, niacin is not good for everyone; there are many patients who report a variety of unpleasant reactions: stomach ache, burning sensations in the skin, persistent itching, headache, mood depression, and mental dullness. In a few cases I have seen hives occur, and, while niacin usually relieves allergic symptoms such as hay fever and asthma, I have seen occasions where it seemed to make the allergies worse.

These may be extreme cases, but it is one reason why megadose treatment should be done under the watchful eye of a physician, preferably one who is experienced in, or at least sympathetic to, orthomolecular principles. Allergic reactions from the use of niacin also support my theory that niacin may actually work to stimulate the anti-inflammatory system. I have seen relatively low doses of niacin cause generalized vasodilatation (red skin and a warm feeling). But at higher doses the flush response no longer occurs. We can assume that the large dose exhausts the body's supplies of whatever chemicals produce inflammation, or else that the body responds to the inflammatory effects of niacin by producing more of an anti-inflammatory substance. My experience supports the latter assumption.

Recently a new class of hormones of considerable importance has been discovered. They are called prostaglandins; among other things, they act as anti-inflammatory agents. In cases of high fever, it has been noted that schizophrenic symptoms of patients clear up temporarily. Prostaglandins are released by fever, just as they must be by the generalized inflammation induced by niacin. Much more remains to be learned in this area; however, we are already able to use the knowledge we do have to relieve the suffering of many patients with schizophrenia, particularly if they are treated before normal personality development is interrupted and damaged too badly.

Breaking the Dependence on Drugs

Recent research has shown that the prescription tranquilizers Valium and Librium interact with nerve cells at the same receptor sites in the brain as does vitamin B_3 (niacin in its amide form). This research, sponsored by the manufacturer of these drugs in search of the biochemical mechanism responsible for the activity of tranquilizers, also showed that less than 1 percent of ingested niacinamide reaches the brain. Doses required to activate nerve cells in lab animals are equivalent to megadoses of 25 grams (25,000 milligrams) per day in human beings. This may explain why large doses seem to be necessary in treating mental illness and certainly supports the theory of megavitamin therapy.

I predict that some day soon an improvement in vitamin B_3 chemistry will replace prescription tranquilizers with a new class of supervitamins. They will not have the potentially dangerous side effects of tranquilizers, such as drowsiness and addiction.

What are the prospects for other drug replacements? The human brain is quite sensitive to changes in body chemistry, and variations in diet are known to affect moods and appetites. Thus, sodium and potassium are known to produce increased energy and muscle tone; calcium and magnesium are natural tranquilizers and muscle relaxants; zinc and manganese are mild aphrodisiacs; copper can be either a mental stimulant or irritant; and iron is sometimes a mental stimulant or irritant and sometimes an antidepressant. Vitamins are less obvious in their immediate action because the brain is stabilized by means of an active vitamin transport system that keeps brain levels of vitamins intact, even when shortages may exist elsewhere. That is, the brain has first priority. By the same token, the amounts of most vitamins that can get into the brain are limited to the number of carrier molecules. Thus, a 40-fold increase in serum vitamin C levels is followed by a mere 2-fold increase in brain vitamin C. While these relationships have not been studied thoroughly enough, it appears that the brain is protected against starvation or gluttony in a reasonably healthy body.

The apparent difficulty in stimulating the brain by even massive doses of vitamins made me, at first, quite skeptical about the use of nutrients in psychiatric treatment of my patients. It always seemed that drug treatment was quicker and stronger. Then I realized that undernutrition may well be a chronic condition in some patients.

If undernutrition is prolonged, even the protein structure of the brain is not immune. Since memory formation depends upon synthesis of nucleic acids and proteins in the nerve cells, severe malnutrition is associated with impairment of intelligence in children and memory impairment in adults, both often permanent. I saw devastating harm done to a patient after his 40-day "therapeutic" fast. Brain damage, memory loss, paralysis, and arthritis—all permanent. I was aware of a number of cases where peculiar dietary practices eventually caused schizophrenic changes in behavior and perception. My own observations confirm that extremely dangerous undernutrition can accompany a prolonged and overzealous adherence to the "macrobiotic diet." The brain is more vulnerable to diet than one would think.

At nineteen, Jennifer T. became convinced through her reading that a fruitarian diet would "purify" her mind, body, and spirit. After six months, her weight had decreased from her original 125 pounds to 80 pounds and suddenly she became psychotic and epileptic. When she came to me, tests showed she had used up almost all of her vitamin B_{12} reserves, and undoubtedly other essential nutrients were also severely depleted by her limited diet of apples, pineapples, bananas, and berries. She also had an enlarged liver and considerable edema suggesting deficiency in protein as well. By luck, rather than the skill of her previous doctors, who had never seen such a case, she survived. Two years later, however, she still had not recovered her vitality nor mental power.

In another instance, brain damage resulting from a dietary extreme proved to be reversible. Chuck C., a nineteen-year-old marine, had graduated first in his class of 120 recruits and was promoted to duties that placed him in competition with men twice his age and above him in rank. To make matters worse for his self-esteem, he was short. To compensate, he went on an aggressive body-building schedule, working out and jogging long distances every day. He took on extra-duty assignments and went with less sleep than usual. To maintain himself at peak condition, he chose not to eat greasy foods at the mess hall but adhered to a strictly vegetarian diet. Unfortunately, his vegetables were nutrient-depleted by remaining on the mess hall steam tables and, since he was stationed at an island post, the nutrient values of the produce were greatly reduced in transportation as well.

A computer analysis of his diet, which I made later, showed 1650 calories per day with below-RDA levels of the amino acid methionine, which is hard to get in a vegetarian diet. He also had low levels of magnesium, calcium, and several B vitamins. Overactive, he was working off 2000 calories a day above the usual 2000 one would expect a man of his size to expend; it was no wonder he lost 30 pounds in two and a half months. Not surprisingly, he finally collapsed in a state of mental and physical exhaustion. What was surprising was that medical personnel in charge of his case interpreted his condition as schizophrenia. They had had no experience to help them identify the cause as malnutrition, nor could they understand his unsuccessful attempts to eat once he was in the hospital. The more he would eat, the more he would vomit. This was diagnosed as *anorexia nervosa,* an inability to eat because of a nervous condition, rather than as a symptom of starvation! When he was finally able to keep his food down, he was believed to be eating compulsively, for his appetite was prodigious. Vitamin and mineral supplements were never included in the treatment program, neither to relieve a brief episode of mental dullness and confusion nor to reverse his malnutrition. Fortunately, he was brought home and given vitamins by his family; he fully recovered from his "schizophrenia" in a matter of weeks.

How Megavitamins Also Help in Less Severe Cases

We saw in Chapter 6 how large doses of vitamins A and C have proved successful in cancer cases, and in this chapter I have shown how B vitamins, some amino acids, and various minerals can often be successful against brain damage and severe mental illness. How about the less sensational problems of depression and anxiety?

Consider Ezra A., who had been unmotivated in school until his 16th birthday. Suddenly he had a new-found self-esteem and an urge to prove himself. At any rate, his grades improved dramatically in his sophomore year and he got involved in sports for the first time. He began to trim down his weight and to drive himself in physical conditioning. Suddenly he fell apart with crippling anxiety. He couldn't even get himself out of bed in the morning. When he did go out of the house, he found that almost every situation made him unbearably nervous. He was fast becoming a recluse and his frantic mother called on several doctors looking for relief. Psychotherapy didn't work because *Ezra was reluctant to talk*. He just felt too nervous to function.

After a glance at his dietary survey form, I could see there wasn't much I needed to talk about, either. He was deficient in just about everything, especially calories. He had been trying to get enough nutrients for growth, intellectual challenge, and physical conditioning on one meal a day—impossible! Then, when he became disabled, he was so upset he wasn't eating at all.

With a little reassurance and encouragement about the cause of his troubles, he was persuaded to try a wholesome diet plan, which included much-needed vitamins and minerals in large doses and some simple health rules, as described in Chapter 13. Ezra recovered without a second visit!

Dr. Carl C. Pfeiffer has reported excellent response to the use of large doses of zinc and manganese in many schizophrenic cases. Those of us in the Academy of Orthomolecular Psychiatry have confirmed this observation many times over. In many cases, patients are poisoned by excess copper from drinking water, due to copper pipes, and occasionally from indiscriminate taking of vitamin pills. Zinc and manganese are prescribed as a natural antidote to copper excesses. A large increase in copper is found in the urine after such treatment. Zinc and manganese are also of benefit in pyrroluric cases, because pyrroles remove quantities of zinc and manganese from the system by magnetic bond, taking the minerals along for the ride when the pyrroles are excreted in the urine. By restoring the minerals with dietary supplements, one can relieve the symptoms of irritability and dysperception, even though the pyrroles may still be excessive.

In the treatment of depression and of insomnia, Dr. Pfeiffer observed that zinc-manganese treatment improves sleep and has a calming effect. Many patients report that with vitamin B_6 and zinc supplements they begin to have normal dreams for the first time in years. (If the dreams become excessive or disruptive it is usually helpful to reduce the zinc and B_6 intake.)

Dorothy M. was a particularly challenging case. She was sent to me by a colleague who was unable to help her with her severe depression: it had been hanging on for almost a year. At sixty-five she had finally had enough of a 30-year marriage to an alcoholic and abusive husband. While the divorce was a relief, the stress of making her decision took its toll. To make matters worse, when she found a warm and considerate male companion, he was unfortunately impotent. After our third consultation there was still no medical diagnosis for her depression, insomnia, and lack of appetite and energy.

Then, as I reviewed her symptoms, I was suddenly struck by her mention of one symptom in particular: loss of taste. Despite the fact that the blood test for zinc and the level of zinc in her hair were within normal range, on the strength of this clue I treated her aggressively with zinc supplements. In three days her sense of taste began to return and with it her appetite. Within two weeks her depression was clearly on the way out and within a month she was herself again. *Sick people need more than the normal amount of nutrients.*

Now the problem that remained was that her friend was sexually inactive. She was aware of his bad health habits: poor diet, heavy smoking, and a bit too much alcohol. He wouldn't listen to her, however, and refused to come with her to a consultation and she was unhappy about this—but not depressed. A few months later, however, he was so impressed by her improvement that he tried her vitamin supplements on his own. This is not something I would recommend, but when she asked my advice for him by proxy I couldn't resist giving her some general hints. It worked! One therapy—two happy people.

After I became involved in nutritional approaches to medical problems, it wasn't long before I realized that the patients who came to see me as a psychiatrist were the same patients who were going to my colleagues, the internists, GPs, allergists, and gynecologists. *Only the diagnostic labels were different.* When my patients presented symptoms that covered multiple systems and fit into no simple diagnosis, I had formerly diagnosed depression or anxiety. But, as my patients began to report dramatic improvement after nutrient therapy, and after I could see with my own eyes the remarkable change in appearance of so many people, I realized that my patients were without a doubt deficient in their nutrition. However, the deficiencies were seldom severe enough to fit into the textbook descriptions of deficiency diseases.

Doctors have not been trained to recognize these mild to moderate levels of deficiency and they are difficult to diagnose. In fact, doctors are taught that these preclinical or subclinical deficiency states do not exist; therefore they are not diagnosed. But the fact is, if there is a shortage of almost any nutrient, the first symptom will be loss of energy. When physical energy drops we feel it as fatigue. When mental energy drops we find ourselves unable to concentrate or sustain motivation. In any case, when there is fatigue or loss of well-being we find any nutrient substance is vital to our health, for "a chain is only as strong as its weakest link." By the use of optimal doses—and this may mean megadoses in some cases—we can usually strengthen those weak links in the body chemistry.

The Nutrition Prescription of Megavitamins

• Recognize the dangers of certain megadoses, especially vitamins A and D
• Check for a niacin overdose in cases of problems with infection
• Increase doses gradually to learn your reference points
• Consider the application of megavitamins particularly in cases of mental disorders, where they were first successful

15

The OC Diet:
Read Your Body

The September 1978 meeting of the Orthomolecular Medical Society was a challenging confrontation for me with our honored guest, Nathan Pritikin. Pritikin is well known for his prescription for longevity and his innovative clinic, then at Santa Barbara: the key to his program was, and is, a Spartan, low-fat diet. Although I came to the question-and-answer period of his presentation with some strong opinions of my own, I was in no way unsympathetic to his views—and no one could argue with his results. Despite the thorough documentation in his presentation and in his best-selling books, however, I had reservations about *why* his diet/exercise system worked, and therefore about what its long-term effects might be. I suggested to him that, by cutting down protein and fat and especially all refined carbohydrates, he was lowering the load on the body's system and increasing the level of micronutrients. "It's not the absence of fat," I said, "but the presence of micronutrients."

He immediately replied with gracious candor, "I never thought of that."

No medical answer, of course, is so simple; everything is a matter of emphasis. In the effort to sell books, however, doctors and publishers alike cater to the understandable desire of readers to "keep it simple." The dieter is constantly on the lookout for an easy answer, the miracle food or pill that will "burn off pounds effortlessly," and the Sunday supplements are where the faddist looks for dietary solutions. It's precisely because the body is such a complex organism that any number of outlandish and contradictory diet schemes actually work to some extent and have rationales for their success. High-fat, low-fat, calories-don't-count, carbohydrates-don't-count diets: they all work for some of the people, some of the time, for some reason or other.

The diet that I'm going to present on the following pages is something of a summary of the message of this book: *know yourself*. Know your biochemical differences and find just the right nutrients to support them; this is the orthomolecular approach. The diet I've alluded to throughout this book, therefore, is not a prescription of what to eat, but a method of discovering your biochemical self. Once you do that, your body will tell you what to eat.

The OC, or orthocarbohydrate, diet fits the image of a popular diet because its basic principle is easy to remember. It has one rule: find your *right* level of carbohydrate intake, and your cravings for other foods will fall into place. Why is carbohydrate the key? First of all, carbohydrate is so important to the functioning of the body that the body can manufacture it by itself from fats and protein. Some 60 percent of available protein can be turned into carbohydrate in the body, and 10 percent of fats. We know what the body requires of protein: about 1 gram for every 2 pounds of body weight (2.2 pounds is a kilogram). And we know that we need about 15 grams, or 1 tablespoon, of unsaturated oil a day for essential fatty acids. But we *don't* know the body's need for carbohydrate in any such terms. It seems logical that, if the body can make the carbohydrate it needs from protein and fats, there is a minimum requirement but great *danger of overconsumption*.

In formulating the orthocarbohydrate diet, therefore, I simply extended the basic concept of orthomolecular medicine—the right nutrients in the right amounts. Perhaps excessive carbohydrate throws the metabolism of the body out of balance, by excess stimulation of insulin and other hormones. Whatever the reasons, it quickly became obvious that finding the right carbohydrate level was clearly helpful to my patients in more ways than weight loss. Primarily, the OC diet restored a certain balance to their general functioning, as registered by an overall feeling of well-being.

Like any diet creator, by the way, I too can offer you some startling and tantalizing facts; perhaps these will serve to motivate you further:

• You can lose weight faster on a 1,000-calorie, low-carbohydrate diet than on a total fast.

• You'll gain more weight from eating three meals than you will from eating the same amount of food in more than three meals.

The Key to Self-Knowledge: Ketones

Before we come to these and other ramifications of carbohydrate intake, let's see how ketones allow us to determine our ideal diet.

Ketones are mild acids, a sort of reserve fuel released from burned fats for survival under conditions of starvation. When we go without food for even a few days our bodies begin living off our stored fats, and these release ketones. Ketosis is thus the state that exists when we're burning stored fats. It is the key to weight reduction, for it can be measured with a simple drugstore kit that detects chemical changes in the urine.

You may have heard about, or experienced, the sensation of improved well-being and absence of bothersome hunger in the second or third day of a fast. This feeling is probably due to another chain of reactions set off by the release of ketones: they inhibit the release of insulin and the stress hormones. Thus blood sugar becomes more stable and hunger is calmed. Without the exhausting effects of stress and irritability of nerve cells, anxiety is reduced. In ketosis the brain cells are calmed down enough to prevent epileptic seizures. It's been established that during ketosis the electrical activity of the brain, as measured on an electroencephalogram, improves in regularity and intensity. Ketones, being acids, also tend to sterilize the urine against infection and even dissolve certain types of kidney stones.

From all these glorious reports, one would assume that ketosis is the state we should aim for whenever possible. In fact, Dr. Atkins' popular diet is based on ketosis produced by a very low carbohydrate intake. Even without reaching ketosis to the point where ketones appear in the urine, insulin activity is reduced and the formation of fat in the cells is slowed. For many people, this is exactly what the doctor ordered. But there's a rub: no matter what the doctor orders, there are individual differences in the ability to tolerate the ketosis. More than half the patients I have introduced to the OC diet experience fatigue and mental dullness at the onset of ketosis. Some want to give up at once, even though they've been told of the benefits that can be expected in a few days. As I mentioned in the previous chapter, lean people in particular have a poor tolerance for too low carbohydrates in the diet. Dr. Tom Bassler, editor of the American Medical Jogger's Association newsletter, claims that a good measure of whether you should continue such a diet is how well you can keep your sense of humor. If you're overweight to begin with, the chances are you'll be able to smile through four or five days on less than 30 grams of carbohydrates. Above this level is a transition point, what Dr. Atkins calls the "critical carbohydrate level," for at 60 grams of carbohydrate a day most people no longer are in ketosis. Two-thirds of my patients find that this level is associated with feelings of well-being. It is optimal.

Isn't this the point of diet, after all? Unless you're being treated for outright obesity, shouldn't you feel your best when you're getting the proper kinds and amounts of food? This is my basic criticism of the general use of either the Atkins or the Pritikin diets, unless they're used for specific medical indications. If they cause distress they're self-defeating. Secondly, when people feel worse as a result of extreme diets they're *not likely to remain on them* very long. That is, they will run to some other extreme instead of trying to find an accommodation between their feelings and their ideals. Such is the lesson of extremism of every kind.

Another factor which has added to the confusion over carbohydrates in the diet is that we use the word rather loosely. When Dr. Seale Harris first discussed the problems of low blood sugar in 1924, he set broad guidelines for treatment: low carbohydrate and high protein. Unfortunately, this has been translated by well-meaning doctors into anything but a low-carbohydrate program. Some anti-hypoglycemia diets advise the taking of orange juice and fruits as snacks, two or three times a day. I was amazed to find one hospital diet sheet, claiming to be a 60-gram carbohydrate program, without the snacks taken into account! The result: twice that amount. By contrast to a low-carbohydrate regime the average American consumes about 300 grams—almost ¾ of a pound. It makes a big difference when changes are made in carbohydrate intake to levels between 30 and 120 grams.

Some nutritionists have reported good results against hypoglycemia with a *high*-carbohydrate diet! Paavo Airola, for example, has been a convincing popularizer of a low-protein, low-fat, high-carbohydrate regimen. How can this be valid in view of the insulin mechanism I've just explained? Again, the confusion results from a misunderstanding of carbohydrates. In the form of complex starches found in grains, seeds, and root vegetables, carbohydrates behave differently in the body. They are digested so slowly that they avoid signaling the release of insulin: they

don't increase the blood sugar level sharply the way refined carbohydrates do. Perhaps we should give these complex carbohydrates another
name.

Which anti-hypoglycemia diet is better? We come back again to the
question of individual differences. Neither low nor high quantities of
carbohydrates are better *in the abstract*. Some people can't use the
Seale Harris guidelines because, even stepping up their meals to six a
day, as he recommends, they find their blood sugar dropping between
meals. Most hypoglycemics can sustain their sugar levels for three
hours, and so suffer no symptoms as long as food is available at those
periods. Some hypoglycemics are better off on the Airola-type diet, but
others are unable to digest grains well and so must resort to a low-
carbohydrate program. In severe cases, for example, wheat intolerance
is characterized by intestinal gas, cramps, diarrhea, and malabsorption.
I've noticed headaches, mood depression, and mental fogginess in many
of my patients after they ate wheat products. Unfortunately, the same
people who are prone to hypoglycemia tend to be allergic to wheat; thus
the low-carbohydrate diet is by far the more practicable answer to their
hypoglycemia.

I've gone into this seemingly technical point in some detail to emphasize the importance of finding a good measure of when one's carbohydrate level is ideal. That measure is ketosis and a little self-awareness.

Dieting to Feel Better, Dieting to Lose Weight

Most of us can lose weight gradually going on a diet that's good for us;
but in some circumstances a drastic loss of weight is the first goal. This
requires a different approach. In either case, you should start with the
following one-week program that is designed to establish your right
level of carbohydrates for optimal well-being. Once you have determined that, you can move on to the OC Weight Loss Program.

This preliminary diet requires only normal food, and if you wish, you
can use a "ketone stick" to determine precisely when you are in a state
of ketosis. (You can buy a supply of ketone sticks at any drugstore.
They are something like strips of litmus paper and change color depending on the presence of ketones in your urine.) If you follow the
suggested diet carefully, you can tell the results without testing your
urine.

The basic idea is that, after reaching ketosis, you gradually increase
your carbohydrates day by day and notice your changes in mood. Unbe-

lievable though this may seem, the changes can be enormous. I predict that even if you are already well nourished you will be able to pick the day you feel best with ease.

You will notice that, unlike other diets, in the OC program you need not pay attention to amounts of protein and fat to any precise degree. The goal is to limit carbohydrates to specific levels. Thus you can boil your eggs or fry them in butter and eat what for you is an "average" portion of meat and fish. The fat content of the meat is of little concern for this purpose. But you will want to avoid flavorings that add up to carbohydrates not shown in this list: fruit flavorings in yogurt, or ketchup, for example. Processed meats contain carbohydrates, but not sufficient to be concerned about.

1. For one week before starting the OC diet, take a complete vitamin and mineral supplement daily. This is simple nutrient insurance.

2. For the first two days eat only average portions of the following:
   - Eggs (any style)
   - Fish or shellfish, fowl
   - Meat of any kind, unbreaded: beef, lamb, pork, even processed meats, including hot dogs and hamburgers, without the buns, of course
   - Two leafy green salads, with one tablespoon of oil and vinegar or lemon as a dressing. With normal portions, each day provides only 12 grams of carbohydrate. Note: water is the only beverage allowed.

3. On the third day, add 24 grams of carbohydrate to the above by adding three portions from the following list, for a total of 36:
   - Cup of milk or yogurt (12 grams)
   - Three slices of tomato (6 grams)
   - Half avocado (6 grams)

4. On the fourth day, add about 36 grams more, bringing the total to 72, by adding three portions from the following:
   - Slice of bread (preferably whole grain) (12 grams)
   - Rice, ¼ cup after cooking (12 grams)
   - Potato, ½ large, baked or boiled (12 grams)

5. On the fifth day, add an additional 36 grams in the form of liquids:
   - Fruit juice, 4-ounce glass (12 grams)

- Vegetable juice, 8-ounce glass (12 grams)
- Fresh fruit, ½ any (banana, orange, apple, etc.) (12 grams)
  You are now at about 108 grams a day.

6. On the sixth day you should double your previous daily intake and observe your reaction to refined sugar, with three portions from the following:
- Candy bar (24 grams)
- Cake, pie (36 grams per slice)
- Ice cream (36 grams per two scoops)
  This is optional, as a test of your reactions, so eat as much as you feel like—or none at all. You are now somewhat over 200 grams—still only two-thirds of the carbohydrates in the average American diet. It's far better, of course, to "go off" your diet with complex carbohydrates, found in starches and grain.

Resume whatever diet you prefer, but think back now about the previous six days. If you wish, keep a log. You should be able to pick the clear winner in terms of your energy level and general feeling of well-being. That, simply enough, is your orthocarbohydrate level.

Your feeling of well-being will prove to be motivation enough to maintain the 100-gram-a-day level, or whatever your ideal carbohydrate intake is.

Notice one important contrast between this plan and the Pritikin diet: fat is allowed in the OC diet, but complex carbohydrates are restricted to the ideal level. It goes without saying that sucrose and refined carbohydrates of other kinds are to be completely avoided wherever possible. One must also avoid overloading even on the best carbohydrates, the complex ones. That's the point, and just about the only point: more carbohydrate *isn't* better.

I have observed that even a 30-gram difference from one day to the next can affect one's mood or energy level. In some cases of mine, the difference was striking. One young man, troubled with a painful duodenal ulcer, felt the symptoms at 120 grams a day; yet even the bleeding stopped when he kept his carbohydrates below 90 grams. Dr. John Yudkin has reported similar results in cases of stomach irritation. In a case of epilepsy, Dr. Darryl De Vivo and his associates at the Washington School of Medicine in St. Louis found that as little as a 1-ounce-a-day difference in carbohydrate consumption was critical. The seizures of a 3-year-old girl couldn't be controlled with anticonvulsant drugs until her carbohydrate intake, including that from fats and protein, was kept within a range of 40 to 73 grams.

Are there any dangers in this one-week test diet? Anyone with kidney trouble, irregular heart rate, or heart disease should be prepared to eat fruit or take a drink of fruit juice if symptoms occur in the first few days of the program. The same goes for anyone, however healthy, who feels unusually uncomfortable. The quick relief of symptoms with only a glass of juice will demonstrate the powerful effects of diet.

The "feeling of well-being" is a necessarily vague description of the goal of this phase of the OC diet. I have heard it described as a feeling of lightness, of not feeling bloated or full, of having more energy, of being able to move around without strain. In the extreme, the opposite is the feeling one gets after rushing, or eating too big a meal. There are also psychological reports: clear-headedness, sharpness, alertness, better moods. Being "at one's best" is a joy. The best way to test your feelings of well-being is to stay at your OC level for a few days, then move up or down the carbohydrate ladder and see what changes. Next, let's see how the same techniques can be applied to the problem of losing weight.

The OC Weight-Loss Program

Regardless of when or how you try to lose weight—no matter what the pill or type of food or ratio of fat-protein-carbohydrate—there are six basic facts about gaining and losing weight that must be taken into account. I ask you to examine those facts and then see if the orthocarbohydrate method isn't the best and safest way to reach your dietary goal.

1. The only safe and lasting way to lose weight is to burn your excess stored fat, not your protein.

2. When fat is burned it's converted to heat energy and ketones, just as a piece of wood burns and produces heat and smoke.

3. Micronutrients fuel the body chemistry and so are necessary for effective burning of fats, just as tinder is necessary for a fire.

4. In a total fast, micronutrients aren't readily available for the burning of fats.

5. More energy for the burning of stored fats is provided by polyunsaturates than by saturated animal fats in the diet.

6. The larger the meal, the higher the proportion of fat that is stored.

There are several interesting and helpful conclusions to be drawn from these dietary facts. Why are many small meals better than a few large ones? Fat absorption and fat synthesis are increased up to 40 percent in the digestion of a large meal, because the body deals with a large intake at one time by increasing the amount of enzymes that convert food to fat. In Chapter 3 I referred to the work of Drs. Leveille and Fabry on the connection between "feasting" at infrequent times and obesity. It's interesting to note that in nature animals that nibble don't become obese.

There are several micronutrients that are essential to the burning of fat. When pantothenic acid is in short supply, body fat is burned at only half its normal rate. Similarly, B_6, the amino acids, and the minerals manganese and magnesium are critical in the burning of fats. It's not surprising, therefore, that the burning of fats actually slows down during a fast; in addition, at the low energy level of a fast it's easier for the body to burn its tissue protein than its fats. The body begins to cannibalize those proteins to get the essential amino acids it needs.

An important corollary to the first fact stated above—that weight is lost effectively only by burning stored fat—is that water loss or gain can be highly deceptive. All of the "miracle" claims for fast weight loss are based on water loss. Hormonal factors cause tissues to retain or lose water, up to 12 glasses of water a day. When you consider that two glasses of water weigh more than a pound, you can see why "mysterious" weight losses of 6 or 7 pounds overnight are possible.

How can you tell, then, if your weight loss program is working? Again, *ketones*. These by-products of burned fat are solid evidence that fat is being burned and weight is being taken off. And this is where the ketone sticks (Ketostix is their commercial name) can be of great help in a weight control program. The Ketostix strips turn a pink or purple color when placed in urine containing ketones. Over the weeks or months of your dietary program you will know that you're burning fat, even though the scale or your waistline may tell you nothing. This can be encouraging enough to keep you going even when you might think you aren't losing weight.

We're now ready to consider a weight-loss program in its specifics, based on the OC diet, supported by adequate micronutrients, and tested by Ketostix.

Step One: Start with the OC "feel-better" diet of six days, with these variations: Make sure your micronutrient supplements are complete and take twice a day during the week before the diet as well as during.

Your supplement label should have at least these values listed, which are the current RDA values. Be sure to read the label, because not all products match these RDA values. Where additional supplementation is needed, it is noted:

Vitamin A: 5,000 units
Vitamin E: 30 I.U.
Vitamin D: 400 units
Vitamin C: 60 mg
   Take an additional 500 mg separately.
Vitamin B_1: approx. 2 mg
Vitamin B_2: approx. 2 mg
Vitamin B_3: approx. 10 mg
Vitamin B_6: approx. 2.5 mg
Pantothenic acid: 20 mg
Folic acid: 400 mcg
Vitamin B_{12}: 6 mcg
Biotin: 150 mcg
Calcium: 800 mg
   You will probably need a separate supplement to obtain this amount.

Magnesium: 350 mg
Zinc: 15 mg
Manganese: 5 mg
Iron: 10 mg (20 mg if there is blood loss due to menstruation)
Iodine: 150 mcg
Chromium: 1 mg
Selenium: 50 mcg
Potassium: generally not in a multivitamin pill; 2,000 mg each day should be taken in a separate supplement. (With enough potassium in your diet, you can use salt freely to make up for the depletion that occurs in ketosis)

There are also some adjustments you should make in the menu of your OC week:

• Among your carbohydrates, be sure to include 2 cups of salad greens and 2 tablespoonsful of raw bran *daily*.
• Limit your proteins to about 60 grams—that is, 3 ounces of fish, fowl, or organ meats, or a cup of low-fat cottage cheese per meal.
• Take 3 teaspoonsful of safflower oil a day (corn, soy, sunflower, and cottonseed oils are acceptable) in order to assure your supply of essential fatty acids.

You may drink tea or coffee during your diet, in addition to water. (In a prolonged low-calorie program, caffeine is known to delay possible symptoms of hypoglycemia).

• I recommend against low-calorie soft drinks, for two reasons: 1. Though they may have only a slight carcinogenic risk, they definitely irritate the stomach and bladder; and 2. They undermine your behavioral conditioning by fostering your taste for sweets, which you know isn't in your best interest. Substitute bottled mineral water.

Step Two: After your modified OC diet week, in which you've established the experience of ketosis and of an agreeably low level of carbohydrate intake, you may want to try a one- to three-day fast, water, vitamins and minerals only. It's a powerful way to initiate weight loss and make a psychological commitment. Even though much of the weight loss in this period may be due to loss of water, the effect on your morale and resolve can be all-important. Ideally, after three days you will have accomplished this purpose and you can gradually return to the diet of your optimal carbohydrate day, as established in the first week.

Step Three: You will be better able to continue to burn fat, as indicated by evidence of ketosis, if you step up the energy level of your body. This means exercise—not necessarily running or jogging, but briskly walking wherever possible (up stairs and to the store instead of taking elevators and the car), never sleeping more than eight hours, and staying uncomfortably cool whenever possible. Drinking ice water and shivering occasionally both cause you to burn up lots of calories!

Step Four: If you intend to lose more than 20 pounds or stay on this program for more than three weeks, ask your physician—*in advance* —for an opinion on the following points: 1. Are you in good health from all normal indications? 2. Does your blood test show a tendency to high uric acid? (If so, sudden weight loss can cause a gouty arthritis.) 3. Do you have a good balance of potassium, sodium, magnesium, and calcium? (If not, the danger is in physical weakness, headaches, muscle twitches, spasms, and irregular heartbeat.) A special word about potassium: the 2,000 milligrams I recommend at the start of the program are difficult to get except in a therapeutic dose by prescription from your physician. Tablets available in health food stores are less than a fourth the dosage. However, the use of a salt substitute, available at the supermarket, may be adequate. A teaspoonful of Morton's Lite Salt or Lawry's salt substitute, for example, provides 1,000 milligrams of potassium.

The Ketone Mechanism

You should be interested in the chemical changes that take place in a prolonged dietary reduction or fast. The more you know about how your body is functioning during that time, the better you will be enabled to "listen" to it for important signals about your health. For, in the final analysis, only your own body can prescribe the ideal program for you to follow.

Make no mistake about it: weight loss comes only from burning more calories than you take in. Protein is hardly stored at all, except as vital tissues; carbohydrate is stored as glycogen, but only in a one- or two-day supply. Fat is the real energy storehouse of the body. But the fat molecule is larger than the carbohydrate and must be burned in stages before it's reduced to carbon dioxide and water. The intermediate stages include the ketones.

Normally we excrete only 20 milligrams of ketones in the urine each day, too little to measure. But this amount is multiplied as much as a thousand times in a near-fast, and this chemical change is easy to detect. The Ketostix will turn pink and then purple as the level of ketones increases. If your scales show a weight loss over several weeks, and you're not in ketosis, only one thing can be happening: you're burning your protein reserves instead of fat. The liver holds only a small reserve of amino acids, and when these are not replaced by eating protein, the body must digest its own tissues. The result of prolonged protein malnutrition of this kind is permanent deterioration in skin, in muscle, and in some internal organs, including the brain. Thus the importance of the ketone measurement in a weight-loss program: to prevent drain of your protein reserves.

By itself, ketosis isn't dangerous; I've referred to it as the normal defense against starvation. But ketones may indicate dangerous conditions, such as the lack of insulin in diabetes. In the case of diabetes, the body is burning its fat and protein for fuel, for without insulin carbohydrate cannot be utilized.

The achieving of the ketosis state may be less difficult if you substitute bran for some carbohydrates. Bran not only contains significant amounts of trace minerals but also stimulates activity of the intestines. Bran also assures increased surface area for the normal bacteria of the gut to grow and so increases bulk and speeds elimination. All of these factors contribute to a feeling of fullness and to faster, more healthful weight loss.

You'll have to obtain raw bran flakes at a health food store; they're not the same as commercial bran cereals. Put 2 to 4 tablespoons in a glass of water and drink it before *one* of your small meals. To assure the presence of plenty of healthy bacteria, you may wish to add a tablespoon of acidophilus bacteria culture (also available at a health food store) to each glass of flakes.

From time to time I stop to remind myself that this simple chemical mechanism of carbohydrate metabolism, micronutrients, and fiber has been fully understood only in our generation. Nothing has fascinated me more as a doctor, nor given me more pleasure, than the chance to apply the wonders of orthomolecular medicine to cases that would have been given up as hopeless only a few years ago. A case I recall with particular satisfaction—it occurred early in my career and helped lead me to full appreciation of the orthocarbohydrate diet—involved almost every factor discussed so far in this chapter.

Marianne W. had had a difficult time of it from her childhood to when she stood before me, at fifty-eight years a troubled, fatigued, over-weight woman who desperately needed to remain active and healthy. She had suffered from allergies all her life and was now developing arthritic pains in her hands, dangerous because she had to continue her art career to support herself and her invalid husband. She was nutrition-conscious, taking liver, yeast, and kelp tablets as well as various vita-mins. Her diet showed no serious deficiencies, at 150 grams of carbohy-drate and 2100 calories a day—with one exception: an intake low in calcium and high in phosphorus. This could affect the allergies and ar-thritis, as calcium is involved in the activity of nerves, muscles, and glands. Yet there had to be more at fault than this.

These are some of the things that turned up in my customary proce-dure of physical examination, glucose tolerance test, and hair analysis. There was some recession of her gums, possibly as a result of chronic calcium loss. White spots on her fingernails suggested other mineral deficiencies, particularly manganese and zinc. A lack of acid in her stomach might account for some of her deficiencies, because acid is nec-essary for the absorption of minerals, especially calcium. Even though her lowest blood sugar level in the glucose tolerance test, 57 milligrams per deciliter, was only marginally below the norm, she experienced a spell of depression and tearfulness at the lab. Low manganese was de-tected in the hair analysis. Finally, it came out that she had avoided salt for years to support her husband's fight against high blood pressure.

The last clue is something that I've seen repeatedly in my practice: an anti-salt regimen that can account for low stomach acid. It's true that perhaps 10 percent of the population can't handle salt because of hy-pertension. For the rest of us I advise heeding the taste buds, which are a good indicator of our salt needs if we pay attention (and aren't addicted to begin with). In short, I advise patients to salt food not just for taste but for effect. In Marianne W.'s case the effect was quite impressive: with the restoration of salt to her diet, her leg cramps cleared up and her fatigue lessened almost at once. Vitamin supplements with manganese gave further relief. A moderate dose of niacin cleared up her allergic symptoms, for which she had been taking antihistamines for years. The niacin consisted of 500 milligrams twice daily; a mild flush reaction followed, stimulating the anti-inflammatory mechanisms of her body to suppress oversensitivity to dust and pollens.

With all of this her gastric acid was still low and her weight excessive at 165 pounds for her height of 5 feet 6 inches. With her full cooperation I started her on the OC diet. The results were eye-opening for both of us. From ketosis on the second day, at which time she was listless and irritable, she easily progressed to the choice of her "right" day. This happened to be the fourth day, at a low level of about 50 grams of carbohydrate. To help maintain that level, I substituted raw bran flakes for 12 of the grams. Within a month she lost 15 pounds. With the bran her diet was so comfortable that she asked me one day, "This is so great—how do I stop losing weight?" The ease of her weight loss was closely related, of course, to the clearing up of her other symptoms. Three years later she was a different woman from the one who first came to my office: allergy shots, pills, and worries about her livelihood were things of the past.

Nutritional Education—the Easy Way and the Hard Way

There is always a section at the end of every diet book that deals with *maintenance.* This is, of course, the real test of a diet. In spite of all the promises about "taking fat off and *keeping* it off," however, this seems to me to be the weak point in all the well-known diets I've come across. For the fact is that a diet is, above all, an educational program; and if a diet consists only of some extreme—low fat, high protein, whatever—it can't possibly teach a life-long nutritional approach.

The OC diet, on the other hand, is personalized, basic nutrition. To continue it into the second and third month and beyond, one need only remember what happened in that first week. There's no need for a drastic shifting of gears, for the OC diet contains no gimmicks.

But one word of caution. From time to time a nutritionist comes to the defense of the American restaurant diet as being adequate if not ideal, and repeats the absurd claim that protein deficiency is nonexistent in this country.

The fact of the matter is that it is hard to get adequate amounts of the essential vitamins and minerals in our everyday diet, let alone in restaurant food. Our cravings may become so strong that we make up for poor-quality food by increased quantity. I am convinced that many people overeat in a desperate search for nutrients that are hard to get in the American diet: calcium, magnesium, chromium, selenium, copper, zinc, manganese, and vitamins, such as folic acid, pantothenic acid, and pyridoxine in particular.

The wish to reward oneself may be a wish to survive after all. But both of these motives may conflict with the wish to be thin. In extreme cases self-starvation can result. Even in successful cases, motivation and self-discipline are important. One of many patients fought his way from 350 pounds down to 175. The OC weight-loss diet has helped him to maintain his weight for eight years—a rather unusual accomplishment, according to all studies of obesity. Here is what he has to say about his triumph over obesity:

> I have had to look neurosis in the eye and face real pain. If your appetite is strong, as mine is, it is like a strong compulsion. There is pain every time I sit down to eat and tell myself to diet wisely. For eating is, to me, a way of taking my eyes off the pain behind it, the problems that push me to eat. Giving up satiety is like coitus interruptus. But I have learned to value a new kind of pleasure: heightened energy and self-esteem. I have learned to do something with the increased energy: I swim half a mile a day and put my energy into exercise. I walk more, I do more. I don't tolerate boredom. When I feel weak and tempted toward food, I call a friend or leave my apartment and take a walk. The urge passes. But I feel more than that I have avoided something: I have created something positive in myself.

He has learned to tune in the new feelings of well-being generated by his now healthier diet and to use the energy so gained in a healthier and more active lifestyle. I urge you to give your body a chance to experience this sound dietary program for two weeks. Find out what the various foods and food balances do to influence your feelings. Learn to heed the signals that the OC diet will make clear, and you may never have to open another book on nutrition or diet.

The Nutrition Prescription of the OC Diet

• Try to establish your best level of carbohydrate intake as a means of improving your general well-being

• Use the OC diet as the safest way to regulate and lose weight

• Insure adequate micronutrients during the diet and your feeling of well-being will indicate your correct carbohydrate intake

16
Foods and Guidelines for Responsible Self-Care

The great French chef Paul Bocuse was invited to Los Angeles a few years ago to prepare a special dinner—at $100 a plate—for a local charity. The gala affair received much advance publicity, and on the morning of the big day a reporter was dispatched to M. Bocuse's hotel room to get a preview of the menu. The chef responded, "I don't know what I'm going to prepare—I haven't been to the market yet."

That we are startled by such an answer is an indication of how we have taken the art of eating and stood it on its head. As it happened, M. Bocuse, with the reporter in pursuit, walked to the nearest fish market and selected the freshest catch, red snapper, and then to a produce market for the vegetables in season. Sampling some California wines, he decided the reds were the best indigenous product, and that evening he presented his guests with a red wine sauce and a Cabernet Sauvignon to go with their snapper. Meanwhile, in the fashionable restaurants of the city, gourmets were dining on broiled lobster (from New England), corn-fed beef (from the Midwest), frozen strawberries, canned asparagus, bottled artichoke hearts, and a variety of main courses prepared by a restaurant-supply company and needing only to be popped into microwave ovens. I once ordered waffles in a pancake house and was surprised to be told that they were all out, for all around me people were eating pancakes. The embarrassed waitress explained the waffles were frozen, to be put in a toaster; they had no waffle irons.

The preserving and packaging of food are supposed to provide great advances in the way we eat, and there's no doubt that we do eat better to *some* extent because of *some* forms of food storage. But we have taken food technology to a ridiculous extreme when appearance and package take precedence over food value. The American refrigerator, the size of a small closet, is a symbol of our basest hoarding instincts. The freezer compartment, necessary at most for making ice and keeping ice cream, is crammed with frozen juices, frozen pizzas, and TV dinners. Many fresh vegetables that belong at room temperature, such as tomatoes, are routinely dumped in the refrigerator produce bin. Root vegetables keep quite well without refrigeration. The American homemaker has been conditioned to believe that trips to the supermarket are minimized by filling the refrigerator; the *reductio ad absurdum* of this reasoning is the deep freeze. Presiding over the back porch, garage, or basement, this offspring of the refrigerator consumes a dollar or two of electricity a day in order to hold, and gradually reduce the nutritional content of, huge quantities of beef, pork, or chicken purchased at a "bargain."

The first step out of our nutritional wilderness is to reacquaint ourselves with the idea of proper marketing—that is, of making routine trips to a grocery store or supermarket to find, as M. Bocuse did, the freshest foods of the season. At the end of this book, therefore, you won't find the usual collection of recipes that are considered *de rigueur* in any book on diet or nutrition. Instead of going to the store with a shopping list in hand, taken from the ingredients listed in a cookbook, why not start with the best available food and *then* look up a recipe for it?

What I propose to conclude with, therefore, is a brief résumé of the *principles* of good eating, so that you can then adapt them to your shopping, your lifestyle, and your health needs. You can refer to this chapter from time to time as a practical guide to the common food sources of vitamins and minerals, the effects of these nutrients, and how orthomolecular practice prescribes them.

Basic Principles of Nutrition

I give all my patients a list of the following "rules of thumb"; simple, easy-to-remember rules are worth books full of exact prescriptions.

1. Eat a little bit of a lot of different foods in as many meals a day as you can. This increases your odds of getting the micronutrients you need.

2. Use your tongue to analyze what's in your food: it's better than a laboratory. These are the four basic tastes you can detect. Sweet and salt in excess cloud the taste buds and mislead your natural cravings; bitter may signal toxins or poisons.

3. There are three basic food types; a single food can contain all of these types, or only one or two of them.
   - Protein sources: eggs, fish, meat (also contains fat), cheese, mixed beans, and grains
   - Fat sources: nuts, avocados, cheese, butter, vegetable oils
   - Carbohydrate sources: whole grains, brown rice, potatoes, squashes, vegetables, and fruit
   - Mixed nutrients: milk, cottage cheese, nuts, seeds (supply all three of the above)

4. Count carbohydrates by remembering them in multiples of six:
   - None: fish, eggs, cheese, meat, fowl
   - 6 grams: 2 tablespoons of nuts, 1 cup of leafy salad, 1 cup of berries
   - 12 grams: 1 cup of milk, 1 slice of bread
   - 24 grams: 1 potato, 1 whole fruit, 6 ounces of fruit juice, ½ cup of rice
   - 36 grams: 2 scoops of ice cream
   - 48 grams: ⅛ slice of pie or cake (Think of the above at your next birthday party.)

5. The "megafoods" are whole foods:
   - Vegetables: beans, peas, nuts, whole grains, seeds
   - Animal sources: eggs, sardines, oysters, clams, organ meats
   - Fruits: berries, cantaloupe, apples, oranges, bananas

6. Take a good vitamin-mineral supplement every day for general health protection. Even the megafoods can't provide everything, every day.

7. Avoid poisons—refined sugar, alcohol, tobacco, caffeine, and additives—where possible.

8. Take bran for fiber, *but only once a day*. Excessive bran blocks the absorption of minerals. Acidophilus helps the bran effect.

9. Think of the following foods in relation to the most common deficiencies:
- Calcium: too much meat, not enough milk and cheese
- Essential fatty acids: not enough avocados, nuts, safflower oil
- Folic acid: not enough raw fruits, vegetables, and liver
- Iodine: not enough shellfish, seaweed, or ocean fish
- Magnesium: not enough nuts, whole grains, green leafy vegetables
- Manganese: not enough nuts, tea, oysters
- Vitamin E: not enough whole grains or vegetable oils

10. Eat in moderation: you want balance and the right amount of nutrients, not excess.

Basic Principles of Self-Care

At the height of the Watergate scandal, the Food and Drug Administration proposed that vitamins should be subject to over-the-counter sales restrictions the same way certain drugs are. There was more mail to the White House over this issue than over President Nixon's problems—in fact, the greatest volume of mail in history. Yet vitamin sales failed to rise significantly.

More recently, Dr. Forrest Tennant surveyed a group of 6- and 7-year-old children on the subject of basic health rules. He discovered that they are surprisingly aware of good health practices but unwilling to follow those rules. I find that their parents act pretty much the same way.

Both these cases demonstrate the old truism that thinking isn't the same thing as doing. Before we can begin to take care of ourselves properly, we sometimes have to be frightened or otherwise doubly convinced that our lives are at stake.

Examine yourself *now* with the same questionnaire my patients use; then try it again six months from now.

What counts is the comparison between tests. You're aiming at reducing the total score and at making the greatest reduction in any or all four sections in which you score high.

If you score more than 20 in sections A, B, or D, or over 30 in sec-

Name_____ Date_____

CIRCLE A NUMBER FOR EACH ITEM ACCORDING TO YOUR CONDITION THIS WEEK. ASK YOURSELF:
"HOW MUCH IMPROVEMENT DO I NEED IN ORDER TO BE HEALTHY AND HAPPY?"

ANSWER KEY:
0 = I need no improvement
1 = I need little improvement
2 = I need moderate improvement
3 = I need much improvement
4 = I need very much improvement

1. Job (even if unemployed do answer) 0 1 2 3 4
2. Living quarters 0 1 2 3 4
3. Spouse or lover (even if you have none) 0 1 2 3 4
4. Family.. 0 1 2 3 4
5. Friends.. 0 1 2 3 4
6. Social life 0 1 2 3 4
7. Hobbies 0 1 2 3 4
8. Sex life (even if abstinent) 0 1 2 3 4
9. Religion, philosophy or meaning of life 0 1 2 3 4
10. Ambition 0 1 2 3 4
11. Money.. 0 1 2 3 4   A_____
12. Self-confidence.. 0 1 2 3 4

1. General health .... 0 1 2 3 4   How healthy and happy do you expect
2. Physical energy .... 0 1 2 3 4   you should be?
3. Resistance to infection or ability to heal.............. 0 1 2 3 4   (Rated on scale 0 - 100%)
4. Sleep... 0 1 2 3 4   _____%
5. Appetite, digestion or bowel function................... 0 1 2 3 4
6. Skin, lips, gums or tongue 0 1 2 3 4
7. Breathing, cough, heart or blood pressure............... 0 1 2 3 4
8. Joints, spine, aches, pains or headache................. 0 1 2 3 4
9. Allergy, hayfever, asthma or eczema 0 1 2 3 4
10. Sex function or menstrual function 0 1 2 3 4
11. Mental concentration ability........................... 0 1 2 3 4
12. Memory for recent events .... 0 1 2 3 4   B_____ AB_____

1. Anxiety or nervousness.................................. 0 1 2 3 4   How healthy and happy are you now?
2. Muscle tension or restlessness...... .... 0 1 2 3 4   (rated on scale 0 - 100%)
3. Indecision .... 0 1 2 3 4   _____%
4. Worry 0 1 2 3 4
5. Fear or panic... 0 1 2 3 4
6. Anger or temper outbursts............................... 0 1 2 3 4
7. Guilt or shame 0 1 2 3 4
8. Resentment or hostility 0 1 2 3 4
9. Jealousy or envy.. 0 1 2 3 4
10. Loneliness 0 1 2 3 4
11. Withdrawal from people or seclusiveness 0 1 2 3 4
12. Boredom or meaninglessness or not caring............... 0 1 2 3 4
13. Depressed mood or low spirits 0 1 2 3 4
14. Over-elated mood, too excited or high 0 1 2 3 4
15. Impulsive behavior or doing before thinking.......... ... 0 1 2 3 4
16. Daydreaming 0 1 2 3 4
17. Putting things off or avoiding goals 0 1 2 3 4
18. Irritable, jumpy or easily startled 0 1 2 3 4
19. Medication dependency.................................. 0 1 2 3 4
20. Alcohol, tobacco, marijuana or narcotics (underline) .... 0 1 2 3 4   C_____

1. Mental confusion 0 1 2 3 4
2. Mind dulled, slow or blank 0 1 2 3 4
3. Thoughts racing or repeating 0 1 2 3 4
4. Thoughts too loud...................................... 0 1 2 3 4
5. Feeling unreal or strange. 0 1 2 3 4
6. Feeling inferior 0 1 2 3 4
7. Feeling mistrustful or suspicious .... 0 1 2 3 4   CD_____
8. Feelings deadened, no feelings.. .... 0 1 2 3 4
9. Feeling hopeless about self or life .... 0 1 2 3 4   _____
10. Hearing voices, seeing visions, hallucination,.................. 0 1 2 3 4
11. Suicidal ideas or self-destructive urges................ 0 1 2 3 4
12 Homicidal ideas or destructive urges .... 0 1 2 3 4   D_____

ExOoSL 1 /8 Copyright R A Kyhst M D

tion C, it's time to make some changes right now. If your problem is in section A, you may have social disappointments that can affect your health. You may wish to explore ways of getting more satisfaction from your work, your relationships, and your lifestyle. This is not directly related to nutrition, of course; the point is to separate those factors over which you have great control from those that may be difficult to change on any short-term basis. But even here change is possible, through efforts to improve your life situation, self-esteem, and your motivation.

If section B is a problem area, a good vitamin supplement may be all you need—or some changes in your diet. Deficiencies are the most common cause of physical symptoms.

If section C scores high, anxiety and depression are significant problems. The nutrition prescription for these symptoms is better timing of your intake of food and adjustment of your carbohydrates. See the OC diet in Chapter 15.

Dysperception and schizophrenia may be indicated by high scores in the final section, D. These symptoms often respond favorably to megadoses of vitamin C, B vitamins, or supplements of magnesium, zinc, and manganese.

Here are some further examples of self-treatment for specific problems, which I offer not as a do-it-yourself guide but as an indication of the power of food in healing:

- Diabetes: the B vitamins and chromium, with yeast a prime source
- Arteriosclerosis: vitamins B and E, and minerals magnesium and selenium as contained in wheat germ
- Bowel cancer: fiber and vitamins A and C, in green leafy vegetables
- Multiple sclerosis, Guillain Barré syndrome: safflower oil for linolenic acid
- Sexual disorders: minerals, zinc and manganese, with sardines and oysters as excellent sources
- Alcoholism: the B vitamins and magnesium, plentiful in liver, nuts and green vegetables

I have had occasion throughout this book to discuss examples of the above in some detail. Here are some lifestyle recommendations, worth mentioning even though they are not central to my theme:

1. Avoid oversleeping. There is a daily rhythm in each of us that is coordinated with the activity of hormones. Oversleeping also allows the buildup of histamines in the body, and so can aggravate allergies.

2. Eat according to your personality; let it guide you in leaning toward food types that support your personality. Extroverts need protein (more eggs, fish and meat) to build up catecholamines (the adrenal hormones). Introverts need extra carbohydrates for their calming effect.

Anyone who exercises heavily needs extra potassium and magnesium as contained in melons, fruits, vegetable soup and nuts. Why are some people "night people" and others most alert at daybreak? If you start the day sluggish, you can balance out your day by taking extra protein. If you're a fast starter, take more carbohydrates for tryptophan, the precursor of serotonin, the brain's natural sedative. Similarly, you need more carbohydrates in the evening if you tend to be an insomniac; and if you finish the day fatigued, boost your proteins then. If you feel you need a tranquilizer, remember that the body's natural tranquilizers are prostaglandins, which are activated by niacin, niacinamide, and vitamin C.

These rules alone are worthy of a book. Don't be afraid to take an active role in self-care. When I was in medical school, the saying was "he who has himself for a doctor has a fool for a patient." But that was back in the days when medical advances were made chiefly in the form of new and powerful drugs. There is no question that in dealing with such potentially toxic molecules as penicillin and cortisone it was folly to treat oneself. This has all changed as far as nutritional medicine is concerned.

Are there dangers in mega-nutritional self-care? Yes, a few. All bottles of pills should be kept safely out of the reach of children. Vitamins A and D are the only known dangerous vitamins. Iron, copper and selenium in overdoses are also toxic. But the danger of toxicity of nutrients has been overstated, in my opinion.

What about synthetic versus natural sources of vitamins? The general rule is always to try to get natural vitamins in natural sources, because foods may contain vitamins as yet undiscovered. A synthetically produced vitamin may be lacking some still unknown trace factor. However, the amount of natural vitamins in a 500-mg pill is necessarily less than in a regular portion of yeast, wheat germ or liver. Therefore, synthetic vitamins are needed. For example: there are strong indications that our optimal need of vitamin C is in excess of what our present diet can provide. For a gram of ascorbate, you'd have to eat about ten oranges. Synthetic vitamins provide this at low cost and without excess calories.

It is not easy to know if a vitamin is made entirely from natural sources or how much from synthetic ones. For example, vitamin C in pill form may be mostly synthetic, even if the label indicates rose hips, acerola, citrus fruits, or green peppers as the source. Various B vitamins are derived from yeast, a natural product; if a chemical name or no source is indicated on the label, it's synthetic. Vitamin E is particularly hard to classify. If the chemical name "d-alpha tocopherol" has an "l" added after the "d," it's synthetic. Is it worth making these distinctions? All other things being equal—yes. Any vitamin made from a natural source may contain more than the vitamin named, just as a vitamin obtained in a whole food contains much more, of course, than a single nutrient.

The great advantage that nutritional therapy has over other types is that it requires work on the patients' part. They must learn to read labels and "listen" to their bodies—truly a case of making a virtue of necessity.

The Role of the Orthomolecular Doctor

At one time, the physician was a sort of hero, a protector who came to the rescue at times of crisis. This role will persist to some extent, but increasingly the doctor is playing the part of adviser rather than savior. Norman Cousins' dramatic fight against illness through the power of his sense of humor and his insistence on treatment with vitamin C is a stirring testament to the self-care movement.

Though the role of a physician is changing, I don't feel its importance is lessening. Instead, the doctor is becoming a teacher and a trainer. Dr. James V. McConnell, professor of psychology at the University of Michigan, writes:

The long-term medical cure rate for obesity is less than 10 percent; the behavioral cure rate is about 60 percent. Yet most physicians continue to prescribe pills and fancy diets for weight loss, when what 90 percent of the patients need is encouragement in learning how to eat sanely. These "cure rate" data have been reported in dozens of scientific journals for dozens of years. Yet just a month ago a man I know informed me that his doctor told him, "You are too damned fat. If you don't lose weight, you're going to die, and it will serve you right." Needless to say, the man became so depressed that he went on an eating jag.

So a good part of the training role of the new doctor is in motivation, as well as in evaluating the facts of a patient's lifestyle. I see my role in motivation as one of getting the patient involved from the very start. So I employ all sorts of paperwork (such as the lifestyle questionnaire mentioned above). Consider the Diet Survey and Medical Symptoms Review that my patients fill out as part of their training. Try it yourself.

Everything is on one side of one sheet of paper, yet it's all there. These are only two of some twenty forms I've developed for various purposes. They succeed in making the patient an active participant and in unearthing and organizing vital information.

Finally, the orthomolecular physician has the important role of ordering and studying laboratory tests to evaluate the body chemistry and investigate dietary deficiencies. Here are some of the important tests that are now in the doctor's command:

1. Blood count, urinalysis and blood chemistry panel remain the mainstays of our evaluation of your general condition.

2. Glycohemoglobin, which measures the extent of diabetes by the amount of sugar bound to the red blood cells. This is the best index of control of sugar in diabetics, and it is easier to perform than the glucose tolerance test.

3. In the diagnosis of hypoglycemia, however, there is no substitute for the glucose tolerance test; nor is there a better way to educate patients to the relationship between their symptoms and their blood chemistry. It's a convincing demonstration to the patient that physical events (fall in blood sugar) have a major effect on the mind and on the emotions.

4. Blood analysis is the best index we have of the possible progress of atherosclerosis. This has been discussed in detail in Chapter 4. A high cholesterol reading (above 250) may be acceptable for certain individuals especially *if* the HDL (high-density lipoprotein) portion of this reading accounts for the elevated level. Otherwise, a high blood cholesterol reading combined with high triglycerides correlates closely with closure of major blood vessels and with atherosclerosis. Dr. Irvine Page recently showed a 95 percent probability of heart disease when both readings were elevated (without reference to HDL). Such a reading is compounded by increasing age.

5. Urine analysis of the 24-hour excretion of vital substances can give a good index of your condition. For example: the 24-hour urinary excretion of such catecholamines as phenyethylamine (PEA) is

DIRECTIONS: Check each symptom that applies at all In the past month.   CIRCLE IF IMPORTANT NOW.

Name _____ Date _____

ALLERGY: □ Foods □ Inhalants □ Additives □ Hydrocarbons □ Medicines □ Asplrln □ Asthma □ Eczema

ENERGY: □ High □ Low □ Normal **APPETITE:** □ High □ Low □ Normal **WEIGHT:** □ Increased □ Decreased □ Unchanged

CRAVINGS: □ Water □ Sweets □ Salt □ Vinegar □ Citrus □ Meat □ Fat □ Eggs □ Dairy □ Alcohol □ Tobacco

HEADACHE: □ Dull □ Sharp □ Stabbing □ Pressure □ Band around head □ One sided
(frequency): _____ per month   (duration): _____ hours
(location): □ Neck □ Back of head □ Temples □ Forehead □ Eyes □ Jaw □ All over head

MUSCLES-BONES: □ Leg cramps □ Stiff neck □ Neck pain □ Whiplash □ Wry-neck □ Sore-aching muscles □ Low back pain
□ Flat feet □ Painful heels □ Loss of muscle power □ Swollen joints □ Painful joints □ Arthritis □ Loss of muscle substance
□ Tired feet □ Tired climbing stairs □ Curvature of spine

SKIN: □ Heal slowly □ Bruise easily □ Dry □ Oily □ Red around nose □ Acne □ Boils Scaly □ Dandruff □ Itchy
□ Red spots □ Brown spots □ Varicose veins □ Scalp hair loss □ Body hair loss □ Seborrhea □ Psoriasis
□ Brittle nails □ Brittle hair □ Eczema □ Excess hair growth Hands usually: □ Warm □ Cold □ Wet □ Dry

EYES: □ Near-sighted □ Far-sighted □ Astigmatic □ Colorblind □ Painful eyeballs □ Halo around light
□ Poor night vision □ Glare sensitive □ Inflamed lids □ Sandy feeling in eyes □ Bloodshot □ See double

EARS: □ Loss of hearing □ Hearing too sensitive □ Earache □ Motion sickness □ Dizzy □ Noises in ears

NOSE-THROAT: □ Sinus trouble □ Post-nasal drip □ Hayfever □ Nosebleed □ Loss of smell □ Strange odors
□ Loss of taste □ Metallic taste □ Bad breath □ Sore throat □ Canker sores □ Change in voice □ Hoarse
□ Lump in throat □ Difficulty swallowing □ Grinding teeth in sleep □ Biting tongue □ Tongue-thrusting

TEETH: □ Toothaches □ Tender to cold □ Cavity-prone □ Soft □ Loose □ Dentures □ Number extractions_____

LIPS: □ Dry □ Chapped □ Peeling □ Split □ Sores at corners   **GUMS:** □ Bleeding □ Infected □ Receding □ Sore

TONGUE: □ Dry □ Sore □ Swollen □ Inflamed □ Split □ Loss of taste Coated: □ White □ Yellow □ Brown □ Black

DIGESTIVE: □ Nausea □ Vomiting □ Belching □ Acidity □ Hepatitis □ Ulcer □ Cramps □ Diarrhea □ Constipation
□ Gas □ Thin stools □ Mucus stools □ Black stools □ Gray stools □ Bloody stools □ Foul-smelling stools
□ Frothy stools □ Rectal spasm □ Hemorrhoids □ Itching anus □ Laxatives:_____ # per month Enema_____ # per month
Food intolerance: □ Wheat □ Milk □ Egg □ Citrus □ Fried foods □ Fats □ Yeast Bowel Movements usually:_____ # per week

CHEST: □ Cough □ Night sweats □ Painful breathing □ Asthma □ Emphysema □ Bronchitis □ Short of breath
□ Green □ Yellow or bloody sputum □ Pleurisy □ Chest pain on exertion □ Irregular pulse □ Rapid pulse
□ Palpitation □ Fainting □ Blackout if get up quickly □ Heart murmur □ High blood pressure

GENITOURINARY: □ Burning urination □ Loss of control of urination (Frequency):_____ # per day _____ # per night
□ Urgency □ Difficulty starting □ Pain in flank □ Kidney stones □ Discolored urine: □ black □ brown □ blood
□ Hernia □ VD □ Lack of sexual information or experience □ Loss of sex drive □ Increase in sex drive.

WOMEN ONLY: Menstrual period_____ days, cycle_____ days. Pregnancies_____ . Miscarriages_____ □ Menstrual cramps
□ Irregular periods □ Nervous before periods Flow: □ Heavy □ Medium □ Light
□ Lack of sexual secretions □ Lack of orgasm □ Vaginal discharge Date of last PAP smear _____.

MEN ONLY: □ Loss of erections □ Premature ejaculation □ Sore on penis □ Pain or swelling in groin

SLEEP: need _____hours; get _____ hours □ Slow to fall off □ Early waking □ Restless □ Disturbing dreams

SPELLS: □ Anxiety □ Heart pounding □ Rapid breathing □ Panic □ Weeping □ Depression □ Elation □ Anger
□ Nausea □ Irritability □ Poor concentration □ Yawning □ Drowsy □ Trance □ Dizziness □ Misbehavior
□ Memory black-out □ Loss of consciousness □ Convulsions □ Weak □ Shaky □ Chills □ Sweats □ Hot flashes
(Spells occur): □ Before meals □ After meals □ If hungry □ If Upset □ Morning □ Afternoon □ Evening

NERVES: □ Numbness □ Tingling □ Burning □ Shooting pains □ Weakness □ Dropping things □ Stroke □ Tics
□ Change in handwriting □ Change in personality □ Loss of memory □ Inability to concentrate □ Tremor
□ Sudden jerks of body or extremities □ Twitching in falling asleep □ Loss of balance □ Clumsiness

MEDICINES USED IN PAST MONTH: □ Antibiotic □ Antacid □ Antispasmodic □ Laxative □ Antihistamine
□ Codeine □ Muscle relaxant □ Tranquilizer □ Sedative □ Sleeping pill □ Antidepressant □ Stimulants □ Diet pill
□ Water pill □ Heart pill □ Thyroid □ Cortisone □ Birth control pill □ Female hormone □ Male hormone □ Asthma medication
□ Inhaler □ Nasal decongestant □ Pain pill □ Anticonvulsant □ Asplrln □ Chelation therapy □ HCG injection
□ B12 injection □ Vitamin □ Mineral □ Other_____

RAKformMSR 1/78 © Copyright Richard A. Kunin, M.D.

an indication of the amount of stress on your hormonal system; and the excretion of PEA (aptly named, one of those acronyms that unintentionally hits the mark) can tell if you are suffering from depression. Surprisingly, you may be depressed and not realize it!

6. You can now have a vitamin profile done on blood or urine to tell you in no uncertain terms what vitamins you lack in your system, and how well you absorb them.

7. The hair analysis for minerals remains the best test we have for deficiencies or excesses of trace minerals and the presence of toxic metal poisoning.

8. A computer analysis of your diet, based on a questionnaire similar to the one on page 236, is a more subjective test; yet I have found it to be highly predictive of possible deficiencies. Such a test is now generally available. I hope it will become more widely used and refined through practical experience.

9. The blood and urine tests mentioned above have many other predictive powers, especially if repeat testing is done. Orthomolecular medicine attempts to observe states of health and changes too small to be called "diseases." This works by comparing all the significant indicators in the blood and urine from one time to the next. The idea is that it is your variation in test results from your healthy period that counts—not comparison of readings to a national norm. Your individual trends are more important than absolute values.

Your physician is your partner, these days, as well as your teacher. You have to learn by your own experience how food affects you and your body. The purpose of this book is to assist you in that study. The quality of your health and of your life depends in large part on how well you learn your own nutritional needs and how to manage them for a lifetime. Only you can provide yourself with "the right molecules" in the right amounts.

MAJOR FOOD SOURCES OF NUTRIENTS

Therapeutic doses of nutrients often cannot be obtained from natural sources alone. This table is intended as a simplified guide to food sources that are readily available and rich in the nutrients discussed in this book—primarily for general maintenance of health and preventive self-care.

Name_____ Date_____

FILL IN MEAL-TIME AND TYPICAL MENU OF YOUR DIET IN PAST WEEK:

Breakfast (_____ o'clock)_____

Snack (_____ o'clock)_____

Lunch (_____ o'clock)_____

Snack (_____ o'clock)_____

Dinner (_____ o'clock)_____

Snack (_____ o'clock)_____

SPECIFY FOOD FREQUENCY (X) OR AMOUNT (#) AS INDICATED BELOW:

Eggs____# per week   Milk____# quarts per week   Specify: ☐ Whole ☐ Skim ☐ Lo-fat ☐ Buttermilk ☐ Kefir ☐ Powdered

Cheese____# ounces per week   Cottage cheese____# pints per week   Yogurt____# pints per week   Ice cream____# pints per week

Liver____x per week   Fish____x per week   Shellfish____x per week   Fowl____x per week   Yeast____# tbsp. per week

Beef____x per week   Lamb____x per week   Bacon____x per week   Ham or Pork____x per week   Sausage____x per week

Hamburger____x per week   Hotdog____# per week   French fries, chips____x per week   Soybean or Tofu____x per week

Nuts____# ounces per week. Specify:_____   Seeds____# ounces per week. Specify:_____   Peanut Butter____x per week

Butter/Margarine____# pats per day   Salad oil____# tbsp. per day   Mayonnaise____x per week   Sour cream____x per week

Bread____# slices per day. Specify: ☐ White ☐ Whole wheat ☐ Crackers.   Cereal____x per week. Specify type:_____

Spaghetti/Pasta____x per week   Soup____x per week   Sweetbreads, brains, kidneys, tripe, oxtail, marrow____x per month

Salad____x per week   Vinegar____x per week   Cooked Veg.____x per week. Method: ☐ Steamed ☐ Boiled ☐ Saute ☐ Baked

Vegetables____total servings per week   UNDERLINE THOSE EATEN AT LEAST ONCE IN PAST TWO WEEKS:

| beet greens | celery | chicory | chinese cabbage | chives | cucumbers | endive | fennel |
| lettuce | olives | parsley | pickles | radishes | rhubarb | turnip greens | sauerkraut | watercress |

asparagus	bamboo shoots	bean sprouts	broccoli	cabbage	cauliflower	chard	collard greens
dandelion greens	eggplant	kale	leeks	mustard greens	mushrooms	okra	green onions
green peppers	red peppers	pimientos	spinach	summer squash	tomato	turnip	water chestnuts	zucchini

| artichoke | green beans | brussel sprouts | carrots | chervil | kohlrabi | rutabaga |
| beets | parsnips | peas | pumpkin | soybean | winter squash |

| barley | corn | hominy | legumes | lentils | potatoes | rice | sweet potatoes | yams |

Fruits____total servings per week   UNDERLINE THOSE EATEN AT LEAST ONCE IN PAST TWO WEEKS:

| avocado | boysenberries | cantaloupe | casaba melon | coconut | cranberries | papaya |
| fruit salad | gooseberries | honeydew melon | lemon | lime | muskmelon | strawberries |

| apples | apricots | blackberries | cherries | dewberries | elderberries | grapefruit |
| loganberries | oranges | peaches | pears | pineapple | plums | raspberries | tangerines |

| banana | blueberries | dried fruits | grapes | guava | huckleberries | mangoes |

Juices____# glasses per week.   Specify: ☐ Tomato ☐ V8 ☐ Carrot ☐ Celery ☐ Lemon
☐ Apple ☐ Apricot ☐ Grape ☐ Grapefruit ☐ Orange ☐ Pineapple ☐ Prune

Coffee____# cups per day.   Sanka____# cups per day   Tea____# cups per day   Water____# glasses per day

Soft drinks____# glasses per week. Specify: ☐ Cola ☐ Lo-Cal ☐ Regular   Tobacco____# per day. Specify: ☐ Pipe ☐ Cigar ☐ Cig'ette

Sugar____# tsp. per day   Honey____# tsp. per day   Candy____# pieces per day   Pastry____# pieces per day

Wine____# oz. per day____days per week   Beer____# oz. per day____days per week   Liquor____# oz. per day____days per week

RAKformDA 1/78 ¶ Copyright Richard A. Kunin, M.D.

Vitamin A: vegetables of all kinds, especially green and yellow color; eggs; liver; dairy products

Vitamins B_1, B_2, B_3, B_6, B_{12}, folic acid, pantothenic acid: brewer's yeast, blackstrap molasses; whole grains, wheat germ, brown rice; liver; most protein sources (eggs, meat, fish, nuts)

Other B-complex Vitamins
Choline: similar to folic acid, plus a major source in eggs
Inositol: fruit, whole grains, nuts, milk, meat, brewer's yeast
Biotin: brewer's yeast, whole grains, eggs, liver, sardines

Vitamin C (ascorbate, ascorbic acid): green peppers, red peppers; broccoli; cantaloupe; citrus fruits, strawberries; cabbage; potatoes; tomatoes; Brussels sprouts

Vitamin D: salmon; sardines; herring; eggs and fortified dairy products; liver

Vitamin E (tocopherol): whole wheat; sunflower seeds; whole grains; leafy vegetables; nuts; vegetable oils; wheat germ

Vitamin K: alfalfa (sprouts); eggs; leafy vegetables; broccoli; liver

Minerals
Calcium: milk and milk products, leafy vegetables, nuts
Chromium: yeast, liver, whole grains, eggs, beans, butter
Copper: liver, seafood, nuts, raisins, molasses
Iron: meat, liver, eggs, fish, poultry, molasses, leafy vegetables, dried fruit
Magnesium: whole grains, green vegetables, nuts, molasses
Manganese: whole grains, peas, leafy vegetables, nuts, eggs
Potassium: seeds, nuts, whole grains, green vegetables, potatoes, bananas, melons, oranges, dried fruits
Selenium: tuna, herring, brewer's yeast, wheat germ, bran, broccoli, whole grains
Silicon: alfalfa, fresh fruit, brewer's yeast, green vegetables
Sodium: seafood, table salt, celery
Sulfur: fish, eggs, meat, cabbage, Brussels sprouts
Zinc: oysters, liver, brewer's yeast, peas, nuts, grains, beans

Index

AUTHOR'S NOTE

*Guidelines from Federal Government stress
vital role of nutrition against disease*

In early 1980, the Departments of Agriculture and Health, Education and Welfare published historic guidelines for Americans to follow in using food as the first line of defense against illness and disease. This action was a significant first step toward reversing official neglect of nutrition by American medicine. Though the guidelines are conservative compared to the recommendations of most nutritionists, they are a welcome acknowledgment of the importance of orthomolecular medicine.

The guidelines note that some forty nutrients are needed for good health. For the first time, official policy now recognizes the link between dietary habits—such as the use of whole foods, complex carbohydrates, and fiber—and protection against the major killer diseases: heart disease, diabetes, and cancer.

A call for moderation, however, isn't nearly enough. Anyone concerned with maximum good health will not be satisfied with less than a nutrition prescription.